The Cochlear Story

CSIRO PUBLISHING Bright Ideas

Dedication

For Adrian and Georgie, my reason for being

(VB)

The Cochlear Story

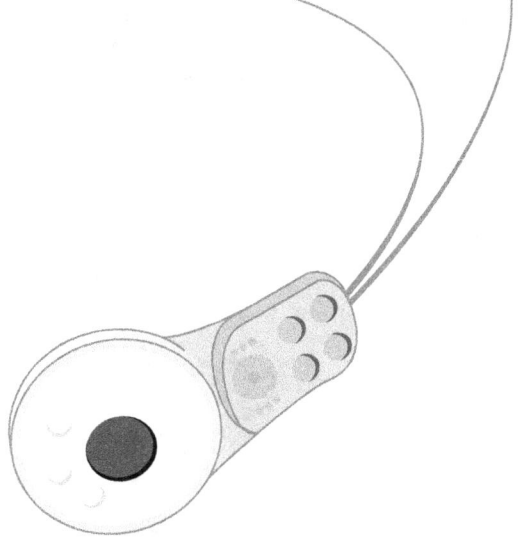

Veronica Bondarew and Peter Seligman

CSIRO
PUBLISHING

CSIRO PUBLISHING Bright Ideas

National Library of Australia
Cataloguing-in-Publication entry

Bondarew, Veronica.

The Cochlear story / Veronica Bondarew and Peter Seligman.

9780643097513 (pbk.)
9780643097520 (epdf)
9780643106840 (epub)

CSIRO Publishing bright ideas.

Includes bibliographical references and index.

Cochlear Ltd.
Cochlear implants – Australia.
Hearing aids – Australia.
Biotechnology – Australia.

Seligman, Peter.

617.88220592

Front cover: illustration by Naomi Dowsett

Set in Adobe Garamond Pro 10/14 and Futura
Edited by Adrienne de Kretser, Righting Writing
Cover and text design by Andrew Weatherill
Typeset by Andrew Weatherill
Printed by Ingram Lightning Source

CSIRO PUBLISHING publishes and distributes scientific, technical and health science books and journals from Australia to a worldwide audience and conducts these activities autonomously from the research activities of the Commonwealth Scientific and Industrial Research Organisation (CSIRO). The views expressed in this publication are those of the author(s) and do not necessarily represent those of, and should not be attributed to, the publisher or CSIRO.

Published by
CSIRO PUBLISHING
36 Gardiner Road, Clayton VIC 3168
Private Bag 10, Clayton South VIC 3169
Australia
Telephone: [+613] 9545 8555
Local call: 1300 788 000 (Australia only)
Fax: +61 3 9662 7555
Email: csiropublishing@csiro.au
Website: www.publishing.csiro.au

Feb26_RP_ILS

Foreword

This fine testimony captures well the struggles and interplay of relations, as well as solutions to engineering and regulatory challenges, that led to the world's first clinically successful cochlear implant, or medical bionics device of any type. It would not have been achieved without the visionary research from the University of Melbourne team, and the creation of a partnership with a vibrant industry.

Once the research by my small team had shown proof of principle, the Australian government gave exemplary help, with financial support allowing the creation of the fledgling company Cochlear Pty Ltd, as part of the larger biomedical pacemaker firm Telectronics.

The engineering challenges faced in taking the design of the University of Melbourne's prototype implant and speech processor to the marketplace should not be underestimated. It was the most complex package of electronics ever placed in a patient. The University provided basic physiological and psychophysical concepts for the design and played a key role in ensuring its biological safety. There were further challenges as Cochlear Pty Ltd had no experience in the hearing marketplace. For that reason staff from the University's Department of Ear, Nose and Throat surgery and from the Royal Victorian Eye and Ear Hospital were essential in providing guidance in clinical matters and establishing important international linkages.

If these difficulties were not enough, in retrospect, it seems miraculous that this enterprise succeeded. At the beginning, 99% of leading scientists said that speech understanding with electrical stimulation of the auditory nerve was not possible, public granting bodies were not supportive and it had to survive on the world stage where severe competition was emerging. Coming from a more protected research environment, I was amazed at how robust the scene was.

I feel sure the collegiality that was part of the University of Melbourne's exciting dream was shared by Cochlear Pty Ltd. Paul Trainor was a fine and ethical industrialist, who did all in his power to transplant people and ideas from the

University of Melbourne, with equanimity, to his new company for this very risky venture. That relationship has continued in different guises and I feel is part of the company's overall success.

Many of the research ideas such as the Multipeak and SPEAK speech strategies, the safe use of high rates of stimulation, protection against the risk of meningitis, bilateral speech processors, bimodal speech processing and the Contour electrode array arose from research at the University of Melbourne, and the staff of Cochlear Pty Ltd have done a superb job in refining the discoveries to make them suitable for clinical practice.

Cochlear CEOs, staff and boards are to be congratulated on developing an internationally acclaimed biomedical industry for hearing restoration, which has had 70% of the world market for 30 years. The present staff under the leadership of CEO Dr Chris Roberts has shown vision in expanding this outreach.

But whatever the financial benefits, the ultimate good is seeing the transformation in the lives of tens of thousands of deaf people worldwide.

Graeme M. Clark AC

Contents

Introduction

A switch is turned on and a little girl's face lights up with pure joy. Catapulted out of her world of silence, she reacts with excitement. She hears her mother's voice for the first time in her young life and her mother cries. The clinician's eyes moisten and a tear gently rolls down his cheek.

The business of bringing sound to over 160 000 people around the world is full of emotion-packed moments like this. But it is a complex business and from initial idea to current reality was nearly 50 years in the making. As always, these great realities start from one person's journey. In this case it could be argued that it started with two people refusing to stay in the comfort zone of current reality and challenging the unknown to do what was thought to be impossible, especially in Australia. But had the story been left to these two extraordinary people, it would have been short. A number of other leaders with very different personalities that underpinned essential leadership styles and skill sets, took the baton and delivered the organisation, its people and its technology to the next level of development. As the baton-passing continued, the number of people catapulted out of their silent world grew exponentially. The amazing benefits that the technology has brought to the recipients, their families, their friends and their communities continue to drive the company and those who work to successfully bring sound to the severely and profoundly deaf.

Australians have long been recognised for their ground-breaking medical research and there are numerous Nobel Prizes as evidence. But as so many commentators have lamented, Australians don't seem to be able to commercialise these outstanding research achievements. The loss to the country's productivity is obvious and well documented. Why is this so? Is it just that Australian entrepreneurs don't have the backbone to take on the challenge, or are there barriers to such development that are too big to overcome? Is Australia doomed to stay in the upstream, research end of the business cycle? This book provides the evidence that the news is not necessarily negative. It tells the story of a number of Australians who have together made an outstanding success of commercialising an Australian medical invention on a global scale. Although there are literally thousands of people who have contributed to the successful process, it could be argued that there was a unique series of leadership qualities that led the company's development at critical stages of its growth cycle. The identification of those stages and the leadership that drove each stage demonstrates what it takes to grow a successful Australian medical device company in the global market. It also provides an excellent model of the possible barriers that can be expected by people proposing similar commercialisation journeys.

The story in these pages focuses on the leaders of the various stages of the company's journey. Graeme Clark was and continues to be a brilliant surgeon and researcher but he certainly operated outside the mould of an academic and respected surgeon. Unlike many researchers, he lobbied government and interest groups for critical funding while managing the disdain of colleagues and students, to achieve the dream. He also understood the need to make the difficult decision to hand over the reins to someone who had experience in the challenges of commercialisation. Many scientific entrepreneurs feel that because they have driven the research, achieved budgetary outcomes in the lab and led a team of researchers they are qualified to lead the commercialisation process. It is their baby, their invention and it is hard to let it go. Clark was not one of those but he did nearly make a critical mistake – he first offered his prototype to an overseas company for possible commercialisation. Fortunately for Australia, it turned him down. If the overseas company had accepted his offer, another Australian story would have been lost to history. It was close.

Clark's commercialisation partner, Paul Trainor, was an outstanding business entrepreneur driven by a vision that he understood very well – how to build global technology platforms in the highly regulated and protectionist country which was Australia in the 1960s. His company, Nucleus, was built on the concept of a central cell nurturing a number of orbiting cells of medical device companies. It was unique at the time and served the industry well. Trainor trawled through university research to pick the gems of scientific discovery. He lobbied governments mercilessly and built his empire on government grants but always with an understanding of the financial essentials that would drive each of the growing number of orbiting companies under the Nucleus umbrella. He often manipulated his staff when it was not necessary, believing that top-grade people work better in tense competitive environments. His strategies, however they were viewed, produced outstanding achievements.

Without Clark and Trainor there would be no invention to commercialise, but without champions in government it is unlikely that any innovation would have taken place. It is all very well to invent in the lab but it is expensive to take that invention to commercial success, to innovate. Champions in government are the third critical element in a successful commercialisation partnership. It is not an exaggeration to say that without visionary champions in the government, there would be no Cochlear Ltd today. At least, not one that is proudly Australian. Commercial development, global market studies, clinical trials and the establishment of global subsidiaries are too costly for a small technology company when it is not earning any income. There were many in government who said it was imprudent to spend taxpayers' money on science fiction, and opposed financial support for the invention. Tens of thousands of people who have escaped their world of silence are extremely grateful to the government visionaries who fought in Cabinet for the initial financial support that would make their hearing world possible.

Engineers and the ear, nose and throat (ENT) surgeons are also critical elements in this story. The highest level of financial support in the world would not be any use without engineers who could create a manufacturable product and without surgeons who could drill into a patient's skull – a patient who may be only two years old – and place the device correctly. The engineers and surgeons championed this innovative industry. Peers and colleagues condemned the idea and said that it was impossible to restore hearing to the profoundly deaf. To this day, some in the deaf community continue to protest against such intervention despite the mountains of evidence of life-changing experiences.

The difference between the groups of engineers and surgeons was, however, substantial. Although the engineers agreed that the challenges were enormous, the drive to overcome the engineering challenges was like having fun and being paid for it. For surgeons the challenge was significantly greater. Surgeons in Australia, the USA, Europe and Japan placed their reputations and careers on the line. If they were wrong, their reputations would be destroyed along with their careers and incomes.

Some truly brave champions were willing to go out on this kind of limb. They were not avaricious. They were not driven by the dollar; the risk did not provide a strong financial return. But they were driven to make a difference in the lives of implant recipients and their families and to ensure that the industry survived. And survive it has, with resounding success.

Trainor understood the need to pass the baton. But although he had little choice, the baton was passed to the wrong team. Therein lies a critical lesson and perhaps one that identifies the real reason why so many Australian companies do not succeed in the commercialisation process. With Trainor gone, the focus changed from the medical to the economic with hazardous consequences. Trainor's umbrella group Nucleus did not survive the change of direction and all the companies under its control were sold or disbanded, except one. One company in the group not only survived but thrived. Cochlear Ltd, under a new leader, Catherine Livingstone, successfully went out on its own. It listed on the stock market with a successful initial public offering, and demonstrated to the world that it is possible for an Australian medical company to become an international leader. Cochlear Ltd is now in the very capable care of one of Trainor's protégés, Chris Roberts. By all accounts, despite a recent product recall, its future remains promising.

Situated below the leadership level are the hundreds, indeed thousands of engineers, surgeons, clinicians, audiologists, marketing experts, lawyers, manufacturing entrepreneurs and financial experts without whom the best leadership in the world would not survive. Where would you put someone like Amitava Sen, who was on the phone till 3am trying to order a critical part that was desperately needed? He is not on the list of heroes, but he was a hero to the person who was sweating on the needed part. There were many situations where people went the extra mile to make things happen. There are thousands of people who should be included in stories like this one, but for practical reasons can't be. Within each chapter there are many stories. It would be excellent to see some of those stories emerge while memories can still recall them.

My thanks go to David Money and Jim Patrick for their assistance and support over the many years required to bring this story to these pages. Peter Seligman, my technological co-author, also deserves thanks for bringing the project back to life after I abandoned it. Without such support there would be no story to tell. I am grateful for the time taken by many people who contributed their time and patience in interviews, making corrections and additions that hopefully produced as accurate a picture of events as distant memories make possible. There are too many people to acknowledge here and many are listed in the appendix. Any misinterpretations are my responsibility.

Mostly this book owes a great deal to Mike Hirshorn, who sadly passed away on 18 November 2011. Tragically, he died without seeing the final product. He was always dedicated to the cochlear project and was a major force behind opening up markets for the implant around the world.

Hirshorn was a most humble high-flyer with a dry sense of humour. His verbal style was non-threatening and gently persuasive. He cared about the fate of people and would rather hear other people's stories than dine out on the details of his own. He was determined to have this story written to record and acknowledge the people who contributed to Cochlear Pty Ltd's success. He also hoped that it would be an inspiration and a guide to scientists and engineers who may want to follow a similar path. It is very likely that without his persuasion, this story about the people who drove the commercial success of the cochlear project would still not have been written.

The extraordinary number of people who attended Mike's funeral attested to the difference he made to many people's lives in his quite unconventional but determined way. He will always be sorely missed.

VB

CHAPTER 1

The beginning: a visionary entrepreneur, Paul Trainor

Paul Trainor was not a happy man as he entered the public gallery of Australia's Parliament House. The public gallery with its dark green leather, dark wooden panels and security guard at the door can be an intimidating place but Trainor was not one to be easily intimidated. He had spent his life taking risks and there was no way he was not going to be heard on this occasion. The public gallery of Parliament House is situated above the chamber housing the House of Representatives. Members of the general public and the press are able to hear and observe the elected representatives dealing with the nation's business, but on no account do they participate in the discussion. They are expected to sit in silence. Guards are at the door to ensure that protocol is observed. They are also there to eject any member of the public who does not behave appropriately and they have done so many times.

The year was 1976 and one of Trainor's roles was to serve on the board of the Industrial Research and Development Corporation (IR&DC) for the federal government. His dissatisfaction on this occasion was based on information provided to him, as a board member, that anyone without university qualifications was ineligible for IR&DC grants. Trainor knew, and his 'bitter bloody experience' (BBE, as he called it) had shown, that innovators were not necessarily academics. He was very much aware that it was not academic qualifications that produced blue-sky research discoveries. Trainor had failed engineering and dropped out of economics at the University of Sydney but had gone on to succeed in running a multi-national company. He was a perfect example of the philosophy that discoveries did not depend on academic qualifications, and it urged him to attend the parliamentary sitting.

At the time the Liberal Party was in power and Malcolm Fraser, having won a double dissolution of the Houses of Parliament, was Prime Minister. His Treasurer was John Howard who, 20 years later, would lead the Liberal Party and become Australia's second longest-serving Prime Minister. John Button sat on the Labor Party side of the House. His education, like Trainor's, was one of BBE. So was the education of many others who were present.

Hushed silences meant little to someone who had left a secure job with his father in one of Australia's leading medical device companies, where he was a director with a good income, to set up his own business in a tin shed. Trainor stood up to speak, much to the alarm of the guard who insisted that he sit down and be quiet. The disturbance caught Howard's eye; on seeing who it was he said, 'Hello Paul.'

A few others looked up and waved. Without hesitation the intruder said, 'There's an issue I want to raise.' Howard turned to the Speaker of the House and asked, 'Can this gentleman say a few words? He is quite a sensible man.' Trainor beamed. He took the comment as a compliment and explained his concern that most developments around the world had been achieved by people who were not necessarily academics. Indeed, in his view most activities were achieved by non-academically qualified people. Trainor had come prepared and gave example after example to prove his point. In a very short time he was getting nods from both the Labor and the Liberal Coalition groups, at which point he ended his speech. Then, much to the relief of the guard at the door, he sat down. It was no surprise to those who knew Trainor that the bureaucrats subsequently changed the wording of the IR&DC Grants Act so that people who were not necessarily academically qualified could receive grants if their cases were eligible.

Trainor was a Sydney boy educated at Marist Brothers College and at St Ignatius, Riverview, a beautiful Sydney suburb situated on the edge of the Parramatta River. He excelled at team sports and was captain of cricket and football, but scholastically he did not achieve so well. He began a degree in engineering, but he did not complete it. As his performance in Parliament House demonstrated, academic setbacks did not constitute impediments to his career. By the 1980s he was invited to lecture and debate at the University of Sydney on international law, world patents and the value of intellectual property, a situation which always gave him a buzz.

Such contradictions were not unusual for Trainor. He was not intimidated by the unknown. He, like the many he would eventually lead, loved challenges, especially by what initially appeared to be impossible.

As a teenager during World War II Trainor went to work with his father, who was originally an optician and who later became skilled in the field of X-rays and microscopic analysis. When he left school he worked in the store in X-ray electro-medical service and attended lectures at university at night. By the age of 30 Trainor was a senior manager in one of Australia's largest suppliers of X-ray, electro-medical, surgical and scientific instruments, Watson Victor Ltd, as well as a director of the public company and its subsidiaries. He was working for a great company with good people, earning an excellent income, but the entrepreneurial spirit directed that he should go out and do his own thing, in his own way. The 20 years spent with his father in the company had given him an excellent education and established the BBE that underpinned and guided his actions towards many of his future achievements in the difficult world he was about to enter.

Throughout Trainor's mid 30s he had kept check of his strengths and weaknesses, calling it 'walking the pebbled beach'. He would go away alone to review the previous year's list of good and bad points to see what he had done to reduce the bad and enhance the good. In 1965, on a pebble beach, aged 38 and with a wife and three children to support, he decided that the time had come to enhance the future and take a risk. With his wife's approval, he sold their prestigious home and moved into a rented house next to the railway tracks. He paid off the mortgage and with the balance started a company aimed at scientific health care.

In the 1960s, Australia's manufacturing base was focused on import substitution, protected from world competition through tariff protection and quota restrictions. Jack McEwen, leader and guardian of the Country Party's best interests, was easily able to drive the concept of high tariff barriers in an environment that feared the spread of communism and potential overwhelming Asian migration from the north. It was an atmosphere that promoted the concept of national self-sufficiency and encouraged highly unlikely industries, such as rice- and cotton-growing that needed huge amounts of water, to become established in a country that suffered from prolonged droughts. Subsidies and other forms of assistance and protection ensured the sustainability of such industries but at a cost that can be measured in opportunity, competitiveness and financial terms. In world parity terms, therefore, Australia was an expensive location. A fixed exchange rate ensured that there would be little change to that situation for some time.

Making international sales was always a difficult challenge. In today's business environment the extent of the challenge confronting Trainor in 1965 is easily underestimated. The 'tyranny of distance' really meant something. It no doubt contributed to the nationalistic, post-war Australian perspective and made overseas communication cumbersome and expensive. The telex machine was the most advanced form of communication technology and any organisation with critical communication requirements was confronted with escalating costs. Anyone who dreamed of creating an internationally significant medical device company based in a country with uncompetitive protectionist policies, no efficient communication systems and a distrust of the foreign, would surely have to be considered foolhardy. An entrepreneurial perspective that saw beyond what was and believed in what could be was a major asset that Trainor brought to his new business. In the next 25 years he kept up with world developments in the high-tech industry – an industry which involves R&D spend rates many times higher than the rates other Australian manufacturers could handle. He began by spending 7% of turnover on R&D when the manufacturing Australian average was 1%. In 1983 he spent $2 million just on travel expenses – more than most government departments would spend on such expenses – and his phone and telex bill reached $1000 per employee. Foolhardy he might have seemed to the casual observer, but there were vision, tenacity and some interesting people skills behind his endeavour.

His business concept went against the trend of the day. He had no faith in the large bureaucratic structures which were then very much the organisational fashion. He favoured separate companies where accountability and responsibility could reside with those executing strategy. The name of his organisation, Nucleus, reflected the concept of a central nucleus, surrounded by cells of activity. These cells would eventually become separate companies, developing markets in a wide range of medical products including diagnostic ultrasound machines, pacemakers, kidney dialysis machines and ultimately cochlear implants, all operating under the Nucleus umbrella.

Having registered the company, Trainor set about devising a positive cash flow and selecting what he called 'A-grade' people who could help develop a profitable scientific service company. To gain cash flow, he entered into service contracts with hospitals and universities to service their sophisticated instrumentation on the basis of a year's contract paid six months ahead, balance on monthly payment. Within weeks of forming Nucleus he travelled to the USA and Japan to establish agencies to meet Australian demand. The initiative clearly demonstrated experience in this industry sector. From the very beginning of operations, Nucleus was focusing on global markets.

Trainor's experience had taught him to negotiate technical and price-sensitive issues as well as terms of payment. He insisted that payment was always 90 days after sight of bills of loading. Such a strategy gave the company time to clear the goods, install the equipment and be paid. Australians love someone who is trying to have a go, and he found that many institutional customers were supportive and some paid before the due date. Some senior government department officials trusted him to the point of saying, 'When you finish up here, your cheque is in the second drawer. I'm off to a meeting.' One time, a reverend mother in Perth gave a substantial order for equipment, involving a very large sum of money. But the shipment was still on the water, it would be weeks before it arrived and at least six weeks before it was installed. This was a particularly stressful time when cash burn was high and there was little in the bank to pay the wages; the team at Nucleus was facing a bleak Christmas with no pay for a month. Whether due to Trainor's negotiation skills, his charm or the Catholic connection, the reverend mother agreed to an immediate 60% prepayment. She said, 'Paul, may God bless you and have a happy Christmas.' Phew! In the beginning, there were many such days. At Nucleus, the families knew that they lived on a cliff's edge. But that was exactly the kind of challenging environment within which entrepreneurs thrive and the A-grade people Trainor chose to work for him were all entrepreneurial in their own way.

He particularly liked the unconventional, being more a lateral thinker than most. He didn't just think outside the square, he thought beyond the horizon. At a lunch on the Mediterranean shores, Trainor pondered possibilities with Chris Roberts who was then Product Manager of Domedica and the Telectronics Greek distributor.

Domedica's principal activity was importing and distributing artificial kidneys which are used in dialysis machines. Domedica had contractual links with a major overseas supplier of those products and acted as the supplier's distributor for Australia and New Zealand. Although Domedica was initially an importer, the mission was always to think of ways to manufacture and export from Australia. Trainor proposed that they export dialysis blood lines (the manufacturing of which had just been established in Sydney) to Greece. The economics of traditional manufacture and export were not favourable but, in an idyllic setting by the sparkling waters of the Mediterranean, Trainor and Roberts sketched a plan to convert shipping containers into portable manufacturing units that could be sent by boat around the world, docking in certain countries, manufacturing a year's supply then moving on to the next location. The concept of converting a jet airliner to a pacemaker manufacturing facility, which could be flown around the world thereby avoiding local import duties in the respective countries, was also a serious idea – but only for the brave. This was unconventional thinking on any scale. Although neither of these ideas was implemented, the thoughts generated other ideas that did lead to implementation and success.

Trainor was good at the big picture, but his key insight was choosing people better than himself in specialty areas such as science and accounting. He saw A-grade people as those with a strong ethical sense and a strong character. An individualist, he was tolerant of other individualists, preferring people like himself that responded to a challenge. He understood that the vision of taking Australian ingenuity to global markets was critically dependent on strong foundations in research and development. This meant finding people who often didn't fit very easily into conventional environments, and letting them flourish in truly creative surroundings.

His choice of people, both in Australia and offshore, depended first on good character and second on their skills. He tried to select people who, irrespective of their qualifications, were top-grade, driven by the challenge not by the money. He hoped they would work 13 or 14 hours a day and sometimes at weekends, and he hoped that their partners would eventually see the merit of this dedication when the financial rewards finally came. Roberts, now CEO of Cochlear Ltd, noted that Trainor could see things in people they couldn't see in themselves. 'That was certainly the case for me', he said. 'Paul had so much more belief in me than I had in myself. That was very motivating and of course you wanted to stretch yourself. Striving for the seemingly unobtainable became second nature. It was one of the best lessons in motivation.'

Providing high motivation, giving autonomy to offshore operations and being flexible in meeting particular requirements was Trainor's modus operandi. With such a team and in such an environment it was possible to schedule work from 8am to 6pm on working days to meet service obligations to pay the bills. After 6pm each evening they busied themselves with critical research and development in keeping with longer-term market forecasts. His exuberance and mental energy made light of the long working week and the company grew in leaps and bounds. By the 1970s, with the firm in its fifth year, Trainor had more than 300 employees and by the mid 1980s it had mushroomed to 1700 employees.

Trainor did not go outside the organisation to find people if he could help it. The Nucleus management chart, starting with the board of directors, was displayed in a public place in the organisation. He included the names of all the people who were currently performing the various roles, and left eight or nine blank squares with no names in them. The chart went all the way through the organisation. He did this so that everyone could see the various companies within the group such as Telectronics, hearing technology (no company name initially), ultrasound technology (Ausonics), scientific & general and so on. Under the company name he listed the managing director or chief executive officer for each subsidiary. Initially, under the company name such as hearing technology there would be a spare box with no name in it. Employees could look at the chart and think, 'Hmm. That position could be okay for me.' This was Trainor's method of encouraging each employee to envision where they might go within the organisation. He would look at an employee and say, 'Okay. You have done all right in that role so why don't we try you out in this role?' Trainor gave everyone the opportunity to rise in the organisation. He also used to say, 'For you to get a promotion it's not up to me. It's up to you to perform well.' But it was not all kind and considerate. He made sure that senior executives didn't entrench themselves and he moved them around regularly and sometimes quite callously, so that no one felt that they were in any one position for a long time. It meant that there were always opportunities for people to come through and they could also seek opportunities for themselves. It was a management style that created a very competitive environment and could be very stressful. Some staff said they were scarred for life. But Trainor continued to believe that hiring A-grade people and putting them into stressful environments worked wonders for the business.

Leslie Farkash, for instance, was an engineer who saw an opportunity on the organisation chart to be head of manufacturing for Telectronics. Trainor had three people in mind, of whom Farkash was one. He gave all three the job of running manufacturing jointly – an impossible thing to do. The idea was to see who emerged as the strongest. Farkash could see potential for improving the manufacturing process. He designed a logistical approach that broke it up so that everyone worked in a little team developing their own output. The design made a very positive impact on Telectronics because the company was able to get products out at a time when cash flow was a real problem. Farkash went up in the ranking for that success, but it was not easy for the two other joint manufacturing managers watch him get the credit on his own. Notwithstanding the competitive stress Trainor created, a lot of people really admired him. It was recognised that if he said something people would believe it and embrace it. Opinion was divided. Some people held him in awe, others thought that he set up unnecessary competition when collaboration would have been better.

Challenging environments can lead to burn-out and disillusionment. A critical element in Trainor's motivation equation was self-interest. He understood that the formula 'A-graders + challenging environment + self-interest = successful outcomes' and set up Nucleus with a profit-sharing plan. Every six months an outside auditor would review the results of budget sales, margins, expenses and before-tax profit, write off bad debts on stock write-downs etc. then take 25% of the pre-tax profit for distribution to staff. Trainor believed in sharing profits as well as striving for them and this was his way of rewarding the extra hours that everyone contributed. As the business grew, he was delighted when some staff received more in annual bonus than in annual salary. But profits were not always equally shared. Trainor had his preferred people who were generally on the medical or engineering side of the business. Those dealing with marketing or financial aspects of the business did not always fare so well.

The basics of setting up and running a medical devices company and the philosophy underpinning the building of A-grade teams were very much developed in the BBE era of Trainor's life. But in 1967, two years after setting out on his own, a particular event epitomised the beginning of his education and knowledge and led to his understanding of what it takes to run a multi-national, multi-channel cochlear implant business. This event led to the establishment of a pacemaker company that provided much of the future funding to pay for the commercial development of the cochlear implant.

In the second decade of the 21st century, Chatswood is a thriving shopping centre and suburb about 10 km north of Sydney, with a very multicultural feel. Its skyscrapers rise above the horizon in a neat cluster of glass and steel, indicating prosperity and growth. A state-of-the-art bus and train terminal transports a thriving mass of workers, shoppers, schoolchildren and commuters throughout the week; on weekends a myriad of families scurry through the maze of retail outlets, buying and carrying their new possessions off to their nests. In contrast to this thriving picture, Chatswood in 1967 was a small, moderately wealthy but very conservative suburb far from any hub of entrepreneurial activity. There, in an unpretentious coffee shop with laminex tables and posters of European locations, Trainor and his new partner George Ferrero met two hopeful would-be entrepreneurs, Noel Gray and Geoff Wickham, to hear a business proposal. That meeting laid the foundation of a multi-national high-technology company long before the term 'high-tech' was ever heard. It also laid the groundwork and company structure upon which Cochlear Ltd would thrive in later years.

In 1963 Wickham and Gray had established Telectronics Pty Ltd, principally to market a device for improving the performance of electronic ignition systems in car engines for people such as Jack Brabham. The project fell on hard times. Wickham was the 'inventor' and Gray was the 'administrator', so Wickham looked for other inventive possibilities. Around 1964, the Royal Prince Alfred Hospital, one of Sydney's major teaching hospitals, offered a prize of £100 to any engineer or other person who could design a working pacemaker. Wickham, it is understood, had not qualified in engineering but, like many without academic qualifications who Trainor related to, had a brilliant and innovative mind. With the assistance of Keith

Jeffcoat, previously a technical journalist on the staff of Electronics Australia, he created the Telectronics model P1, a workable design for a pacemaker. The problem, of course (almost replicated in Cochlear 20 years later), was the shortage of money to develop prototypes to the degree of reliability required for implant in cardiac patients. Having heard that Trainor was becoming a key figure in the medical device industry, Gray and Wickham invited him to the coffee shop meeting to propose that he become a shareholder in Telectronics.

They explained the basic concept of a pacemaker, which was simple enough. If a heart does not receive the regular electrical impulses which cause it to beat, it is possible to generate the pulses artificially and apply them to the heart via attached electrodes. If properly applied, the heart will respond just as it would to the natural impulse. The snag was finding a practical way of doing this. If the pulses had to be generated outside the body, how could they be taken inside the body to the heart? It was tried, but without much success. The obvious alternative was to put all the equipment inside the body, but how could it be made small enough and how could it be powered for long enough to make the idea worthwhile? The development of the transistor, compact high-energy batteries and miniature components were the starting points. Two engineers, Wilson Greatbatch and Ake Senning, working independently in the USA, produced the first implantable pacemakers in 1958. Nearly a decade later, a company in Australia had a workable design that needed support to prove the concept, carry out trials and demonstrate the possibility of commercial manufacture.

At a historic board meeting soon after the coffee shop proposal it was agreed that Nucleus Ltd, the company owned by Trainor (85%) and Ferrero (15%) would acquire a controlling interest in Telectronics Pty Ltd by purchasing 50% of the shares in Telectronics Pty Ltd and gaining the right to nominate the majority of the board of directors. This was completely documented in the minutes of the board meeting in 1967. The new company, in a modest upstairs premises, now had start-up capital of $40 000. It also had some difficulties with the owner of the noodle shop downstairs, who complained about the acid that occasionally dripped down through the floorboards into his shop!

The learning curve provided by the new acquisition rose very quickly for Nucleus. Shortly after acquiring control of Telectronics, the Nucleus Group was sued by

American Optical for patent infringement. It took a while but eventually American Optical won the case and Telectronics was obliged to pay licence fees. Never one to miss an opportunity, Trainor approached Bill Nealon, the American Optical in-house lawyer, to work for Telectronics, which he did. Trainor also engaged Mike Rackman of GRR as Telectronics' US patent attorney. The two men were seriously good A-graders who had essential legal global credentials in patent protection and during the early days Rackman provided critical advice on the importance of registering patents to protect the company's intellectual property. How Trainor managed to get two senior lawyers working for successful US companies to jump ship and join an obscure Australian operation, situated on the other side of the world in a zone not exactly recognised for its manufacturing ability, is an interesting question. Anecdotes tell of promises of first-class travel and of working from home, but those are minor considerations. Could the answer lie in the meeting of entrepreneurial minds and the similarity of drive to meet insurmountable challenges? Whatever the reason, it was a brilliant move that benefited the Nucleus Group for many years. Both lawyers provided consultancy advice to Telectronics in 1994 even after the sale of Nucleus to Pacific Dunlop, although Nealon's contribution may not have been so positive in the final days of Telectronics.

In 1967 Telectronics commenced research into technologies which could allow hermetic sealing of the pacemaker to preclude water vapour penetration and as an interim measure it contracted AWM, a subsidiary of Amalgamated Wireless Australia Ltd (AWA), to develop integrated circuits for the electronics. The early integrated circuits were developed by David Money, a seriously good A-grader, who later joined Telectronics and became the first CEO of Cochlear Ltd. Putting the icing on the technological A-grade cake, David Cowdery joined the company in 1970 and developed a revolutionary hermetically sealed pacer. Telectronics' model P8, released in 1971, was the first pulse generator with a hermetically sealed metal can, giving the company a competitive advantage in the industry. The ability to hermetically seal electronic equipment so that it would not be corroded by bodily fluids was later used by Cochlear Ltd. It was a major reason for the company's success and it has been said that no other company, certainly no other Australian company, could have been successful in the commercial production of the bionic ear.

Trainor sent Lloyd Ferreira to establish US offices in an effort to take over pacer distribution in Buffalo, NY in 1974. He also sent Cowdery to France to establish a factory in that country. When General Electric exited the pacer market in the USA, Trainor negotiated with the corporate giant to allow Telectronics to manufacture the Australian pacers in the old GE premises. 'To do this', he explained, 'we acquired the manufacturing facility of General Electric's pacemaking division, after a long and arduous negotiation. This was achieved but we had no cash for such an acquisition. So when I was flying the red-eye special from LA to Milwaukee (where the factory was) I joined the queue for the john, fell into conversation with a leader of the Wisconsin unions who invited me to have a beer and as a result of a chat he said if you do the right thing by the workers I will have a talk to General Electric. This he did. We negotiated employing five people per month for 10 months so that we were then in a position to introduce our technology into the GE plant and pay GE over two years for the capital equipment required for manufacture, which had previously been owned by GE.' It was the promise of protecting those 50 jobs that got the union to support his proposal.

These developments created major opportunities for Nucleus. By being US-made and working with nationals, the company established networks and distribution chains in the world's largest implant market. It also developed in-house expertise in patent protection and networks with the US Food & Drug Administration (FDA) without whose approval it is not possible to sell medical devices in the US. 'Our strategy in the USA', Trainor said, 'was to ensure that we always complied with FDA standards so that we could not be blocked from the American market. Most countries are sophisticated in standards and effectively use such tactics as a means of trade control, for example DIN standards in Germany, Homologation in France, and Underwriters Laboratory and the FDA in the USA.' With the Nucleus head office in Sydney it was necessary to vest heavy authority in the subsidiaries to ensure swift decision-making within written policy guidelines and in line with budgets. Naturally, monthly reports were made by all subsidiaries but there was – and had to be – frequent, almost daily communication by phone, fax or personal visits. Nucleus strategy also became more sophisticated over the years, so much that market projections for the upcoming five or 10 years were done before developing nursery research projects. In this way the organisation was able to forecast its R&D to market needs, with cost–benefit analysis. As the Nucleus Group expanded it gained additional expertise in each new destination, which could be called on later when it was building the cochlear implant business.

On 31 January 1979, the Australian government announced a public interest grant to achieve commercial development of a University of Melbourne-developed cochlear implant. The groundwork for Nucleus to apply for this opportunity had been set over the 12 years since the coffee shop meeting in Chatswood. Not surprisingly, given its technological and worldwide expertise, the Nucleus Group won the tender to perform a market study and write a development cost plan for commercialisation.

The market study identified sufficient worldwide demand to justify commercial manufacture of the device. Among several contenders, Money was appointed by Trainor as the first CEO of Cochlear Ltd (as it later became known). Money was well aware of the issues facing the company. He had been intimately involved with development of the pacemaker and knew that to achieve and maintain success he would need a reliable product that could be produced fast, with honest claims and at a realistic price. His strategy was to license the intellectual property from the University of Melbourne and, with a team of university and Telectronics experts, jointly manufacture the implant in facilities in Sydney for the final-stage FDA trials. It was the beginning of an extraordinarily successful journey that would change the lives of over 160 000 people worldwide during the next 30 years.

The Nucleus Group continued to grow at 50% per annum and the fruits of R&D, marketing and manufacturing saw new products appear in the market. Intensive-care cardiac monitors, X-ray equipment, pacemakers and the beginnings of the cochlear implant continued to be refined. Many other concepts were on the CAD drawing boards but, as is sometimes the way with R&D, some projects were not cost-effective and/or were impractical. The economy of scale of such specialised products needed a market much bigger than Australia, so Trainor proceeded to establish export systems into other countries. He would call people into his office and, after giving minimal advice, say, 'Here is a typewriter and a pacemaker. Go and open our New Zealand branch.' This strategy worked surprisingly often, and it always made a profit.

Regardless of the location, finance was always an issue. Raising financial support in the USA, France and Switzerland was very different from doing so in Australia because international banks understood the value of innovative R&D and the potential of new medical technology. As the company expanded into overseas markets, so did Trainor's understanding and appreciation of the workings of international finance. When Cochlear Ltd was looking for finance for commercial development in the early days, this knowledge and skill came in very handy.

With the help of Rackman, worldwide patents were generally lodged in most western countries. In subsequent years valuation of intellectual property was also required, and additional A-graders were employed to carry out this important function in a field involving such high technology. Their expertise allowed the company not to be intimidated in litigation with high-worth players such as the US Navy. There was a case that went on for some years and cost over $US500 000, but Nucleus won. When the Navy appealed, Nucleus won the appeal as well.

In the late 1970s Telectronics opened in Japan and gradually gained a good share of the pacemaker market. Cochlear Ltd would later benefit greatly from this initiative. In a country such as Japan with restricted access to foreign products it can be difficult to appreciate the time and cost involved in having medical devices approved by the regulatory authorities. Approval takes many years and millions of dollars. Consequently, the selling price in Japan of such products is a lot higher than the price in the USA and the UK. In the long term it can be very profitable but much patience and perseverance are required.

In keeping with Australia's growing recognition of the need to develop productive relationships within Asia, Nucleus had specialists on staff to build tangible relationships in the region. Nucleus, specifically through Ausonics, was one of three Australian manufacturing companies to be visited by China's Premier Li Peng during his historic visit to Australia in 1992. It took over 10 years, with the company's specialists in China, to build the relationship of trust between the People's Republic of China, the Australian government and Nucleus that allowed such an event to take place. Consequently, Nucleus was honoured, not only with being one of only three Australian companies to be visited but also by the trust of the Chinese government in purchasing its equipment, knowing that the purchase would be supported by the training of its clinical, engineering and service staff in China and in Sydney. Trainor had always followed the strategy of building positive relationships with China even when its political position was not recognised by Australian governments. He made sure that visitors, wherever they came from, would have their personal needs met and were always made to feel at home and welcome in Australia.

Building relationships is critical in growing any business but especially so in the medical devices business, given the diverse personality and professional types that populate the industry. As with the early venture capitalists in San Francisco, Trainor kept a keen eye on research developments in various Australian universities and was able to build valuable relationships to support his business base. He could mix with everyone. If he needed to bow to royalty he would. But if he was with people who wanted to get the facts really quickly, he could be a knock-about bloke. He could be charming and well-mannered or as rough and tough as he needed to be. He certainly knew how to act very professionally. It depended on the occasion. There were occasions when arguments would get quite heated and there were times when he was extremely polite.

Chameleon qualities are particularly useful for nurturing valuable government contacts. Among Trainor's many contacts was John Button who, like Trainor, was a self-made man, having come up through the trade union movement in South Australia. Button's skills were honed over many years and he was a very clever and active politician. He had a vision much like Trainor's and it has been said that they learnt a lot from each other. They saw a lot of each other and enjoyed drinking socially, giving them the opportunity to discuss industry policy, R&D grants and efforts to set up venture capital. Such occasions were not made public. At that time the Nucleus Group received a lot of money from the government in export grants and R&D grants and it was important for there to be no perception of favouring friends.

Despite all Trainor's skills, the responsibilities of Nucleus Group directors and team were growing increasingly complex. Performances in finance, technology and marketing were under constant review. In the mid 1980s sales were approaching $A200 million but a review of long-term goals demonstrated additional financing requirements. Trainor asked, 'Could we achieve our growth in the 1990s without putting the Nucleus Group at risk of a foreign takeover? Could he as the major shareholder continue to block a hostile takeover yet continue to provide the equity for growth?' The answer appeared to be in the negative; the decision was made to select a suitable Australian company to take the Nucleus Group forward. Thus, in 1988 Pacific Dunlop acquired 100% of Nucleus Ltd and its group of companies. Trainor, the founder and key motivator, left the business entirely. He returned a good proportion of the profit from the sale to staff, research and friends.

Hundreds of Australians who worked in Nucleus' hothouse environment had learnt Trainor's philosophy of creativity, innovation and internationalisation. Over the decades since Nucleus, their experience affected the success of a whole raft of Australian companies.

Trainor's achievements were recognised. He won many awards for his daring and innovative ideas, including being appointed an Officer in the General Division of the Order of Australia for service to secondary industry, particularly in the field of medical technology. In June 1984 the Nucleus Group was the recipient of the Governor-General's award for Outstanding Export Achievement. It was only the second time the award had been made since its inception in 1979 and of the six winners at that time, only the Nucleus Group had been twice honoured. Australia's medical device industry remains one of the most successful Australian industry sectors. For this, Trainor deserves to be proud. He is truly the father of Australia's medical device industry.

CHAPTER 2

Also in the beginning: a visionary scientist, Graeme Clark

The entrance to the Department of Otolaryngology at the University of Melbourne (UOM) has Professor Gustav Nossal's words inscribed on a plaque commemorating the success of the cochlear implant in terms that put the achievement into its true perspective:

> *The cochlear implant is the first and only device produced by mankind which effectively restores the use of one of the human senses.*

The Australian driver of research into electrical stimulation to restore hearing for the profoundly deaf was the foundation Professor in Otolaryngology at the UOM, Professor Graeme Clark. He was appointed to the position in 1969 at the very time when Paul Trainor was going through his BBE in implantable devices. It is interesting to note that the learning curves of the two critical drivers of cochlear implant commercialisation were moving in the same direction, at the same time, in the same small Australian market. It was inevitable that their paths would eventually cross and that they would collaborate. The success of that collaboration is attested by listings on the stock market and by the 160 000 people who formerly lived in a silent world and who can now hear birds sing.

The similarities between the two visionaries are many. They both came from and valued strong family connections and the educational environments that provided strong moral codes and leadership skills. Neither man was prepared to stay within the comfort zones developed by others. Both were determined to forge their own destinies in their own way. Like Trainor, Clark gave up a good income and security within private practice. He uprooted his wife and family and began life on a lecturer's salary so that he could research something that, at the time, was thought by physiologists to be impossible. Trainor and Clark both saw not what was, but what could be, and they both intrinsically understood how to choose the best people to help achieve the impossible.

Towards the end of 1966, the year that Telectronics was being introduced to Nucleus, Clark stopped to have lunch in the leafy solitude of the small park adjoining the Royal Melbourne Hospital. He read a journal article while he ate his sandwich. The article was by Blair Simmons and it described the hearing of strange sounds by a person who had had electrical currents passed through wires placed in their hearing nerve. The article made it clear that there was still much to learn before profoundly deaf people might be able to understand speech by electrical stimulation of the hearing nerve. Although the patient couldn't understand speech, the report was enough to excite Clark's interest. Unlike Trainor, Clark's academic qualifications were exemplary. He finished top of his final year in medicine at the University of Sydney then trained as a surgeon, qualifying as an ear, nose and throat surgeon at the Royal College of Surgeons, London. On returning to Australia, he settled into an ear, nose and throat partnership in Collins St, Melbourne and searched for an area to which he could make a contribution. The article described exactly the kind of project Clark had been searching for. It was also an area that was close to his heart. His father, a pharmacist, was hearing-impaired with sensori-neural deafness. He often had to ask customers to speak louder when consulting him about their medical needs, which embarrassed all concerned. Such moments left Clark forever conscious of the difficulties faced by those who cannot operate efficiently in the hearing world. He understood, however, that before he could contribute to the project he would need to learn a great deal more about auditory brain science.

Full of enthusiasm, Clark contacted Professor Bishop at the University of Sydney and arranged to work with Dr Colin Dunlop, who had been appointed to do research in hearing and brain science in Sydney. He gave up his well-paid private practice and moved his very young family from Melbourne to Sydney to take up the low-paid research position. He learnt how to study the hearing pathways in the brain and found working in the department of physiology an enlivening experience. It had people who were established and highly respected scientists and Clark learnt from them what science was about. His time as a researcher provided valuable lessons, among them the realisation that scientists thought very differently from most doctors. They had an overwhelming commitment to discovering new knowledge. Understanding that there were different perspectives within disciplines on the discovery and development of knowledge gave Clark a sound foundation in understanding how to deal with the disparate groups of individuals that he would be required to engage with, in years to come. Most importantly, during his three years at the University of Sydney he became totally committed to continuing the research on electrical stimulation of the hearing nerve, convinced that it could assist in reproducing frequency information to help profoundly deaf people understand speech. Clark returned to Melbourne in 1969 as foundation Professor in Otolaryngology at the UOM and the research experience at the University of Sydney served him well during the next 10 years of ground-breaking research that led to the prototype of what became known as the bionic ear or the UOM cochlear implant.

The invention of the cochlear implant is a muddy story. In a normally functioning ear, sound waves travel from the environment through the outer ear. The sound waves then move on to the middle ear where they cause the eardrum and three tiny bones to vibrate. These vibrations are coupled to the fluid in the snail-shaped inner ear (cochlea) where thousands of sensory (hair) cells are each connected to a hearing nerve. These tiny hair cells in the cochlea change the vibrations into electrical energy in the hearing nerve that sends sound signals to the brain. In the profoundly deaf, the hair cells are so damaged that hearing is prevented.

Profound deafness can be present at birth. Injury or an illness such as bacterial meningitis or mumps can also cause profound deafness. Profound deafness is different from hearing impairment. The latter group can be assisted to hear through the amplification of sound by various means such as hearing aids. Amplification of sound will not help the profoundly deaf to hear but fortunately, although they may have lost their hair cells, most profoundly deaf people still have large numbers of hearing nerves.

The cochlear implant system places electrodes into the cochlea to electrically stimulate the hearing nerves. The question of who invented the system can be divided into single-channel and multi-channel devices, although the division is rather blurred. The origin of the single-channel system is relatively straightforward. It was invented by the French. Regarding who invented the multi-channel cochlear implant, it is necessary to rephrase the question and ask who developed the first multi-channel (as distinct from multi-electrode) cochlear (as distinct from auditory) prosthesis (as distinct from experiment of no benefit to the subject). There appears to be no clear answer to this question, but it was probably also the French.

The first attempt to develop a clinical cochlear implant was made in 1957 by two Frenchmen, André Djourno (an electrophysiologist) and Charles Eyriès (an otolaryngologist). A recipient was implanted with a single-channel device. Unprocessed sounds were transmitted via a pair of coils. The link was transcutaneous; it did not require a break in the skin after implantation. This implant failed after a short time and another device was implanted. After the second device failed, Eyriès refused to implant a third device. He urged Djourno to collaborate with an industry partner to build a more reliable device. Djourno refused to do so because he believed that academia should not be tainted by commerce. Djourno found another surgeon, Roger Maspétiol, who implanted a device in another patient in 1958. The patient was eventually lost to follow-up. Although the recipients were unable to understand speech with the device alone, it did help with lip-reading by providing the rhythm of the speech. Through the lack of an industry partner, the French lost their initial lead in the field.

By 1961, William House, together with John and James Doyle, had commenced work on a single-channel device in Los Angeles. House's work continued in the 1970s in collaboration with engineer Jack Urban. Their implant was also a single-channel device but the speech was modulated onto a carrier of 16 kHz. The device, manufactured by 3M, was ultimately implanted in a thousand or so recipients and paved the way for future clinical development of multi-channel cochlear implants. The House/3M unit was the first cochlear implant to be approved by the FDA for implantation in adults, in 1984.

Blair Simmons, author of the article that stimulated Clark's interest, implanted some recipients with a six-electrode array in the modiolus of the cochlea at Stanford University in 1964. The first subject was an almost-blind man with tunnel vision, which added significantly to the difficulties of testing. The device used a percutaneous (through the skin) plug that enabled the electrodes to be individually stimulated. Recipients could still not understand speech via the device but, importantly, it did demonstrate that by stimulating different areas of the auditory nerve, different pitch percepts could be produced. However, its use was limited as no take-home speech processor was available to recipients.

In 1976, a paper was published on the subject by Paul Pialoux, Claude-Henri Chouard and Patrick MacLeod. In the six months prior to the paper being submitted seven patients had been implanted with an eight-channel device. Although it was reported that about 50% of ordinary words were understood without lip-reading, this was not supported by audiological data in the literature. A group at the University of California, San Francisco was formed at about the same time by Francis Sooy, who recruited Robin Michelson and Michael Merzenich. The group did much basic neurophysiological research in the field. They used an electrode array consisting of platinum balls embedded in a single silicone carrier. Analog stimulation was used. A percutaneous plug was used initially, with the intention of converting to a transcutaneous (wireless) system. However, this development never eventuated. The group at first collaborated with Storz Medical Instruments and the work eventually led to the formation of Advanced Bionics, a current competitor of Cochlear Ltd.

At around the same time, Chouard in Paris was experimenting with a similar device, which importantly used sequential pulsatile stimulation on 12 channels. This did not have the problems of channel interaction experienced by the Melbourne group but the stimulator used a voltage source and thus loudness changed over time with variations of electrode impedance. The group began implantation of its device in 1977 and had treated 60 patients by 1983. Chouard's collaboration was first with Bertin & Cie then with MXM/Neurelec.

Don Eddington at the University of Utah tested a four-channel percutaneous plug device in 1978 with an intra-cochlear electrode array. This electrode had six platinum balls placed 4 mm apart with the best four channels being used. The speech-processing strategy was called compressed analog and it used four bandpass filters. An extra-cochlear return electrode was used. The Ineraid device was manufactured first by Symbion Inc. and later by Smith & Nephew Richards Inc. medical company.

Because of its percutaneous plug, the recipients of the device were useful research subjects for many years.

Another active group was headed by Erwin Hochmair and Kurt Burian at the Technical University of Vienna, Austria. At the time this group used a hermetically sealed glass package developed by PhD student Ingeborg Hochmair. In 1977 Professor Kurt Burian implanted a patient with a multi-electrode cochlear implant. The device failed and no speech processor was tried. By September 1978, a six-channel device had been tried and some open set speech performance was reported. Subsequently, only the best one of four channels was used. After some collaboration with 3M, Erwin and Ingeborg Hochmair eventually moved to Innsbruck and founded the company Med-El, which is still one of the four manufacturers of cochlear implants. The company was the first to produce a behind the ear (BTE) processor, albeit using a single channel only.

Numerous other projects were also under way during this period, in the UK, Germany, Spain, Switzerland, Brazil, Denmark, Belgium and Canada. It could be said that Djourno and Eyriès pioneered the way with the first clinical attempt, House with a successful single-channel implant, Simmons with a multi-channel implant, Merzenich and White with more multi-channel work, Eddington and Chouard with filterbank strategies and John Lilly with an electrical stimulation paradigm. None of these projects, however, was able to restore speech recognition to the profoundly deaf. The achievement of speech recognition was Clark's mission.

The two drivers behind the flurry of activity in the cochlear implant area throughout the 1960s and 1970s were progress in electronic engineering and intensive neurosensory research. It was within this climate of discovery and evolution that Clark began his research. Unfortunately, despite an environment of many new discoveries, his vision was not accepted by his colleagues and his claims were considered to be outrageous. His friend and mentor, Professor Colin Dunlop from the University of Sydney, let Clark know that he was very concerned about Clark's rash claims about bringing hearing to the deaf. He could not understand how Clark could make statements that his breakthrough would be as exciting an advance as heart transplants. Others accused Clark of fabricating his research results on nerve/brain cell connections. The problem was succinctly described by Simmons, who was working at Stanford in California. While attempting to discuss his own implant experiments with prominent researchers in speech coding and auditory psychophysics, he wrote, 'I got a distinct impression ... that most everyone was either incapable of thinking about the many problems involved or would rather not risk tainting their scientific careers.'

Throughout the 1960s and early 1970s (and even to some extent today), the research climate drew a line between pure and applied research and saw them as two very distinct enterprises. But Clark had been trained as a surgeon as well as having a strong research interest. Therefore, although his appointment to the first Chair of Otolaryngology in Australia provided the opportunity to do things his way, he was neither fish nor fowl. He was not a pure scientist and neither was he an applied surgeon. Colleagues complained to the UOM vice chancellor, Sir David Derham, that Clark was wasting his time on experimental work that was leading nowhere. They had expected him to spend more time training ear, nose and throat surgeons, as did professors in North America and Europe. Leading ENT surgeons in Melbourne were deeply disappointed in the inaugural professor and requested the vice chancellor to have Clark removed from his position. Fortunately, this request was not granted.

Although Clark's position was difficult, it helped him to cross boundaries in work that required a multi-disciplinary approach, which meant not adopting a 'pure' research perspective. Clark got excited by neurophysiology then by engineering. Worse still, he practised the surgery and, even worse, tried to get money! It was a new experience and he was well aware that academically he was committing to the wrong track. It was very well known even then that academics were motivated less by commercial outcomes than by the peer recognition of innovative, ground-breaking studies. That was and often remains a very strongly held perspective. Clark, on the other hand, was always fascinated with Louis Pasteur who believed there are only two sorts of research – not 'pure' and 'applied', just 'good' and 'bad'.

Clark's single-minded determination to go against the grain of contemporary thinking was not unlike Trainor's vision of basing a global medical devices company in a country protected by tariff barriers and a nationalistic focus on self-sufficiency. Like Trainor, Clark was determined to succeed and he was fortunate in gaining support from various influential supporters, among them Professor of Ophthalmology,

Gerard Crock, who believed in the value of Clark's research and supported him throughout many difficult years.

The issue of acceptance by the scientific fraternity became urgent, however, when Clark made applications for funding to the National Health and Medical Research Council (NHMRC). He got no help at all: his applications were peer-reviewed and his colleagues all canned them. One time, Clark asked John Billings, chairman of the NHMRC, why the body had rejected a grant application. The reply was, 'You have got to stop putting cochlear implants in the title. You have got to do your research and call it something else because your colleagues are all blocking it.' If the UOM and the NHMRC wouldn't help, then to continue his research into developing a multi-channel cochlear implant Clark would have to find other sources of funding even for such basics as an electrical stimulator unit and rolls of film.

Clark did manage to get funding from various other sources using an interesting variety of means. He took Billings' advice and reworded an application, winning the first and only NHMRC grant he received until after he had proven the concept. The grant meant that Clark could ask research students to work on the project since he at last had some money to buy equipment. He went to service clubs such as Apex, Rotary and Lions Clubs and gave presentations on the importance of his research, receiving excited applause and much-needed financial assistance. The UOM gave him permission to run a public appeal, which brought in trust and foundation money. There was no way to avoid the need to raise money, as only sufficient funding would permit even an attempt at research. The USA gave loads of financial support to R&D and there was close collaboration there between academia, industry and government. In Australia there was no such close collaboration so Clark had to struggle on, searching for cash in what many of his peers thought was a most ungainly manner. Fortunately, he raised sufficient funds to begin the work. He would have loved to have had more money, but he did the best with what he had.

Clark realised very quickly that he could not do the research alone. He had learnt at the University of Sydney that medical students did excellent research and, what's more, they didn't cost any money. They also provided a pathway into various departments through their supervisors. Such access to bodies of knowledge was very useful. Clark wrote to several medical students and invited them to join his project; he was delighted when John Nathar, David Scrimgeour and Harry Minas joined him. Howard Kranz and Aileen Williams with psychology backgrounds and Joe Tong, a graduate mechanical engineer, joined later. By 1972 he had a group of students actively researching whether the stimulation rate of a single electrode would be adequate for speech recognition. They worked closely together and there was a feeling of great camaraderie. They were young and enthusiastic and together they were eagerly discovering new territory.

Although Clark didn't believe that a single electrode would provide speech recognition, for several reasons it was vital to carry out this initial research. In the mid 1970s the single-electrode device being developed in Los Angeles was coming into fashion and scientists and surgeons were advocating that the more complex and therefore more expensive multi-electrode system that Clark was focusing on, would not be needed. Clark considered that he shouldn't embark on expensive development of a multi-electrode implant to reproduce the place coding of speech frequencies unless he was confident that the single-electrode device would not do the job. He needed to be sure, so that he could answer critics and be confident that any experimental studies on humans were necessary and on the right track. He decided that he would rather over-prove his group's results than have someone else prove them wrong. By the end of 1973, he and his small team of researchers were able to prove that a single-electrode implant would not be an effective bionic ear. Their studies also alerted researchers to the problems with percutaneous plug-and-socket models when connecting external electrical stimulation to the hearing nerves. Infection could be passed through the skin. This supported the need for an electronic package that could be implanted under intact skin, although it was more expensive.

But now came the really difficult question. Would a multi-electrode implant achieve speech understanding? Finding the answer meant expensive engineering and being confronted with the need to raise cash again. Worse, the money that had already been obtained with so much difficulty was insignificant compared to what would be required for the multi-channel development.

Clark, like Trainor, had an outstanding level of people skills and was equally gifted in his ability to inspire people from across personality, career, national and social boundaries. After a talk he had given to the Apex Club, he was photographed being presented with a cheque as a donation for his research. Sir Reginald Ansett, owner of Channel 0 (now Channel 10) television station, saw the news item and asked Clark to discuss with him the possibility of Channel 10 conducting a telethon to raise money for the research. The channel was ultimately inspired to run not one but three telethons over a number of years. In an effort to motivate viewers to donate, it showed a 10 minute documentary on the bionic ear. Clark was part of that documentary, adding acting to his already large portfolio of skills. Having to emerge from behind potted plants to repeat lines over and over again with all the appropriate gestures, that he invariably got wrong, left him with a life-long respect for professional actors and directors.

The telethons and accompanying street appeals raised substantial financial resources that allowed the beginning of research into the multi-channel implant. The telethons also gave another valuable resource. The event was opened by the then Premier of Victoria, Rupert Hamer. Other politicians who provided support included the Leader of the Federal Opposition, Billy Snedden, the Federal Minister for the Media, Doug McClelland, the Federal Opposition Spokesperson for the Media, Dame Margaret Guilfoyle, the past Premier of Victoria, Sir Henry Bolte and the Mayor of Melbourne, Ron Walker. The Federal Opposition members were soon in government and Bob Hawke, who was then leader of the Australian Council of Trade Unions, was Prime Minister of the Labor government that followed the Liberal defeat in 1983. Exposure to such a wide audience of leading members of parliament was a very valuable resource in the years to come when Clark was looking to the federal government for financial support.

The development of the multi-channel cochlear implant project evolved through three stages. The first step involved understanding the physiology of how sound was processed by the brain. The second stage focused on the more expensive task of developing an electronic package and an electrode array that could be implanted within the inner ear. The third stage focused on speech-processing strategies and their ability to analyse sound. In 1973 the project had reached the second stage and, without any engineering expertise himself, Clark was grateful that he was able to convince an electrical engineering colleague at the UOM, David Dewhurst, to help design complex circuitry for an implantable receiver-stimulator unit that would stimulate the hearing nerves. This part of the project required a senior electronics engineer but, as always, there was no money for one. Dewhurst, whose interest in the project had been ignited by the telethons and who, like Clark, wanted to work on projects to help people, introduced a postgraduate engineering student, Ian Forster, to do the research for his PhD.

The first telethon raised $87 233, which allowed Clark to pay for an engineer, a computer programmer, a technical officer, electronic parts and some other equipment. He kept a little aside for continuity of staff but avoided telling them how uncertain their future was.

Jim Patrick was the successful applicant for the engineering position, although he never knew how precarious the funding was for the position and how close he always was to losing it. Late in 1974, Patrick was in the process of completing his PhD in communications systems in the Department of Electrical Engineering at the UOM. His job prospects seemed to be teaching at RMIT or doing research in places such as Telecom. Although technologically interesting, the lack of human involvement did not appeal to him. Dewhurst was one of his lecturers and suggested that the research being conducted at Otolaryngology in the medical faculty, for the hearing-impaired, might interest him. Enabling a person that was deaf to hear was quite a contrast to the other type of work options open to him, and Patrick took it.

In January 1975 when Patrick joined the team, Clark had about 10 postgraduate students and a laboratory manager but no one to coordinate the project and be responsible for the engineering aspects. Patrick initially worked on specific projects. He found himself in a small department where everyone was very energetic and there was an extraordinary range of activity. The researchers had huge freedom to set their own hours and it was not uncommon to work seven days a week for 12 hours or more. They were driven by the challenge and the possibilities. It was not unusual for meetings to take place in the evenings on the beach, with windsurfers and partners in tow. Mid-week tennis and table tennis matches were organised, taking on a Wimbledon-competitive tension. The researchers were young, they had vision and they were all driven by the science and the sense that what they did could make a profound difference to patients – their research could make people hear who otherwise might never have heard a sound. That was an incredible impetus.

The research was multi-disciplinary from the beginning. There were researchers from the psychology department, doing animal experiments proving that cats could hear sounds differently when electrodes were placed in different locations in the cochlea. Others were making single-unit recordings, putting the electrode right into a single nerve fibre. Others were working on the spread of current through the tissue. Ian Forster, working under the supervision of Dewhurst, was busy making circuits and Rick Hallworth was thinking about ways of making electrodes with help from Australia's Defence Science and Technology Organisation (DSTO). His project involved depositing thin films of platinum on Teflon and exploring how electrode patterns could be etched into the platinum.

Patrick's job evolved over the next couple of years and he became project manager for the whole project. By 1977, as the time to implant patients came nearer, the critical problem was working out how big the implant was going to be. Clark acquired some temporal bones; these were measured and blocks of wax were cut into different shapes to see if they could fit into the mastoid behind the ear, which was to be the implant site. It was very sobering to see all the electronic circuitry that Forster was designing and compare it to the small space it had to fit into. It didn't look as if it could possibly work.

The initial aim had been to produce an operational benchtop model that could be tested before miniaturising the circuit onto silicon chips. Clark took study leave and went to Europe to pick up ideas on how best to work through the electric challenges and to obtain a good understanding of speech science, so that he could know what information would be important to include in the implant for speech understanding. His trip made him aware of the growing international interest in cochlear implants and the competitiveness of this area of research. He was not concerned, naively thinking that when he returned his group might be able to package the implant and do the first operation. Unfortunately, on his return he found that there was still a lot of work required to complete the benchtop model. With a deep sigh, he accepted that electronics circuits don't always perform to expectations and he would need to be patient until the work was completed.

The solution took 18 months but they did it. By late 1977, the silicon chip controlling the stimuli on each of 10 stimulus channels was complete. Forster had combined the control circuits on a custom-designed Mastermos silicon chip, with one chip needed to control the stimuli on each of the 10 stimulus channels. Ten of these digital chips were assembled onto three ceramic substrates, together with another 35 chip components. Using hybrid technology, the chips were connected by gold wire bonds to tracks screenprinted onto the ceramic substrate. Australia's telecommunications company, Telecom, provided its latest facility and produced the hybrid substrates free of charge, while Hybrid Electronics mounted the components onto the substrates. Working at a microscopic level, Patrick stacked the substrates and connected them with more wire bonds. The electric assembly was tested at high temperatures for a week to screen out any infant failures. It was also thoroughly dried before sealing and tested for helium leaks to prove it was hermetic, following advice from Telectronics. Although not designed for reliability, it worked. Patrick searched catalogues and bought, from a US company, a gold-plated box that was designed to hermetically seal aerospace electronics. He convinced an assistant in the Department of Mechanical Engineering to create a new lid for the box because the stack of hybrids was higher than the height of the box. The sealed box was gold-plated then covered with silicone rubber to form the implantable unit.

The final problem was the intra-cochlear electrode array. Rick Hallworth and the DSTO project were not ready, so the surgeons tried different ideas themselves. One promising concept was to take a bundle of leads, strip the insulation off one lead for the last few millimetres and form the electrode by wrapping the bare platinum wire around the bundle of leads. Although this could be inserted quite well, the design was abandoned when it became clear that the ear would be badly damaged if the wrapped electrode bundle had to be taken out later and replaced with another. Clark was floored. He had advertised that he would be implanting a patient very soon and the thought of putting off the surgery until after further research was not appealing. Clark and his group of surgeons and engineers sat around a table and tried to come up with a solution. Quentin Bailey suggested, 'Why not wrap a band of metal around a silicone tube at each stimulation site?' He later said modestly that, 'My contribution was a one-liner.' What a one-liner! It led to a design that was used in about 40 000 recipients. Having said that, the idea was simple but implementing it was extraordinarily difficult. With Hallworth still in Adelaide, Patrick took up the challenge. Suitable components were available: Teflon-coated platinum wire, 0.6 mm diameter silicone tube and platinum foil, but the very small size of the components meant that construction would have to be carried out under a microscope. The foil electrodes needed to be tightly wrapped to compress the silicone rubber tube so that no sharp edges were exposed. Tiny welding electrodes were ground from tungsten rod, to weld the platinum components. It would be quite a fiddly job and, after Patrick's successful construction of prototype arrays and successful temporal bone insertions, the group was fortunate to find Sue Derham, who had the deft fingers needed for microscopic construction. The banded electrode array had many advantages. It could be inserted and withdrawn without injury to the inner ear and it had a large area of electrodes, so that it had low charge density for safe stimulation of the auditory nerve. It could be inserted without the need for correct orientation, making consistent insertion less dependent on the skill of the surgeon. Twenty years on, an improved and more easily manufactured version was still the most effective and commonly used electrode array.

Clark then turned his attention from engineering to the surgical procedures that would be fundamental to the implant's success. He had designed several necessary operating instruments and had worked out that a bundle of electrode wires could be inserted into the inner ear without the loss of the hearing nerves. The most appropriate place to make the skin incision had been considered with Brian Pyman, who would be Clark's assisting surgeon. They had determined how to drill into the skull to accommodate the package without hurting the facial nerve, which would cause the face to droop or become numb if damaged. In more serious instances, damage to the facial nerve can cause a number of additional problems including pain or paralysis of part of the face. To ensure that they had mastered the surgical techniques, the two surgeons practised the operation on about 50 human temporal bones before carrying out their first operation. To minimise the risk of infection, they adapted a method of operating in a flow of filtered air to ensure that they couldn't contaminate the wound with microbes shed from their bodies or circulating in the theatre. Concerned to produce a reliable surgical procedure that could be followed by other surgeons, they drew up a surgical manual. This manual became the basis for implanting further improved bionic ears.

As engineering of the receiver-stimulator for the bionic ear proceeded, Clark was well aware that it was time to find suitable deaf patients. He would look very silly if, after having promised so many people that implantation would happen, there were no patients who needed the device. However, the telethons had increased public awareness – some people had written to Clark directly and others had approached him through the Australian Association for Better Hearing. He decided that he would initially operate on only a small number of patients even if it meant that the results would not be representative, in case there were unexpected outcomes. Also, because of the controversial nature of the operation, he would operate only on patients who had previously had hearing and who had totally lost their hearing – they had nothing to lose through volunteering. It was important that the patients selected were people prepared to take risks. The implantees would need to be robust in temperament in case things went wrong. They were pioneers and satisfactory speech perception could not be guaranteed, so they would need to be able to accept the fact that this knowledge would help others. They would also have to understand that they would need to visit the research facility several times a week for psychophysical tests and to have their speech processor programmed.

The delays in engineering were fortunate in that they provided time for the first patient to be identified. Rod Saunders came to see Clark in April 1978. He had received a head injury the previous year and his skull had to be opened to stop the bleeding. After the operation Saunders became totally deaf. He could no longer do his job and spent much of his time at home. He had not succeeded at lip-reading. To Clark, Saunders appeared to be an appropriate first patient.

On Tuesday 1 August 1978, Clark left home to do the first bionic ear operation. He had done everything he could to ensure that the operation was a success, including a whole lot of praying. A lot was going to rest on the result of the operation. He had been promising the public so much for five years in exchange for donations. If he failed, his reputation would be destroyed and a lot of people's hopes would be wiped out. The theatre was prepared. The patient was wheeled in, reassured and sedated. The units that would blow sterile air across the open wound were set up and Clark asked for the scalpel. As he pressed firmly downwards while sliding the knife along the planned path behind the ear, he knew without doubt that he was gambling his whole career on this operation.

Family members and staff watched the surgery with bated breath via closed-circuit television. It took eight very tense hours. There was a communal sigh and a sense of relief when the operation was completed and the incision was finally bandaged. The operation was a success but they would have to wait to see how effective the implant would be. For now it was enough to see that Saunders' vital signs, especially brain function, were good. As the evening wore on without drama, Clark finally allowed himself some sleep. He had done all he could. The device was made and implanted and all he could now do was wait and hope for good results.

Four weeks later when the wound had healed, Saunders returned for testing. The team was ready for this moment. Patrick and Forster were ready with the equipment to transmit signals to the implant. Tong was managing the computer programs to control the implant and help Clark to interpret the sensations Saunders experienced. Everyone tried to act as if this was routine, but the anxiety was palpable. On the first day Saunders heard nothing. It was very depressing for everyone to send him home without any results. The same happened on the second visit. Clark spent sleepless nights wondering what could have gone wrong but, before the third visit, Forster discovered a fault in the test equipment that explained the lack of results. The fault was fixed and Saunders heard sounds. All 10 electrodes were working. In an effort to see if he would recognise voicing and rhythm of speech the team played the national anthem, 'God Save the Queen'. Saunders bolted upright, dislodging some of the leads as he stood to attention. There was no doubt that the implant worked. The press was notified and the news received wide coverage in both the national and international press. The stories claimed that because the patient could recognise 'Waltzing Matilda', there was hope for speech understanding.

Although euphoric about Saunders' results, as the end of 1978 approached Clark was again dogged by financial concerns. Programmer John Gwyther went on holiday and when he returned Clark had to tell him that he no longer had a job. It was difficult. Clark had enough money to pay Patrick for another three months. Then there would be no more money. A grant from the Ramaciotti Foundation for $15 000 for Forster's salary was about to expire and possible government funding was still not approved. But the research was not finished. There was still the problem about how to convert the successful speech-processing strategy that had been developed using software commands on a large laboratory computer, into a box of electronic hardware small enough for a patient to wear.

The first speech processor, the subject of a PhD by Rod Laird, used a filterbank to split sounds into their component frequencies and simultaneously stimulate corresponding electrodes. The problem, however, was the volume of the sound. There was extreme and uncontrollable loudness growth. The current to the electrodes could be individually adjusted but, when used together, there was no way to control their loudness. The stimulations of the individual electrodes interacted strongly. Back to the drawing board. What the team did not fully realise at the time was that it was not the filterbank that was the problem, but simultaneous stimulation of a number of electrodes. This has been referred to as the mistake that created a billion-dollar company. The problem was solved by using sequential stimulation, where only one electrode is active at any one time.

About this time, University College London had its own cochlear implant project. It involved a single-channel device and aimed at providing voice pitch as an aid to lip-reading. The project was under the direction of Adrian Fourcin, the voice pitch guru. Fourcin's work revolved entirely around voice pitch and he was the inventor of the Larynograph, a device that depicted pitch graphically to help hearing-impaired people control their voices. Bruce Millar from the Australian National University was studying at University College at the time and subsequently returned to the ANU. He worked as a consultant with the UOM team. With a multi-channel cochlear implant, it would have seemed silly to provide only one speech feature (voice pitch) so the UOM team asked Millar what he considered to be the most important speech feature. He said that it was the second formant, or second resonant peak, of the speech signal. The first formant was visible on the lips and so was not considered necessary, as it was not an aid to lip-reading. Thus the first UOM successful speech-coding strategy was conceived – the second formant was coded as an electrode or position of stimulation in the cochlea and the stimulation rate was used to present the voice pitch. Much psychophysics was done to ensure that the simultaneous presentation of these two parameters did not cause them to interfere with each other.

The concept was strongly supported by the fact that when a fixed-rate pulse burst was presented to different electrodes and the implant recipient was asked to identify the closest vowel sound, he consistently ranked position in the same sequence as the second formant, with more basal electrodes corresponding to vowels with higher second-formant frequencies. This was a key experiment.

Very early one autumn morning in 1979, Peter Seligman was woken by his four-year-old son who said that there was a man on the phone who wanted to speak to Dr Seligman but obviously it was a wrong number because there was no doctor in their house. Fortunately the child had not hung up, and Seligman found Clark on the other end of the phone line. Seligman had approached Clark in October the previous year asking if he could join the research team. Although Seligman was perfect for the job, there was no money to fund any more staff. Clark now informed Seligman that Forster, worried about the security of his job, had accepted an offer to work in Zürich. Did Seligman still want the job? Thus began a 30-year career in a job that Seligman described as 'having fun and actually being paid for it'.

If there was ever a case of being in the right place at the right time, Seligman felt that his arrival at the Department of Otolaryngology at the UOM must have been it. A PhD on hearing in a Department of Electrical Engineering was certainly the right qualification, and six years in industry helped too. By 1979, the Department of Otolaryngology had implanted two patients, Rod Saunders and George Watson, and the work of trying to develop a speech-processing strategy was beginning to bear fruit. The trouble was that talking to the patients required a room full of equipment and Seligman's first reaction was doubt that it could be achieved quickly. He believed it would be at least 15 years before there would be a practical device.

Seligman's doubts were reinforced on attending a seminar held by Patrick at the Institute of Radio and Electronic Engineers, where Patrick showed a graph that horrified him. The tonotopic property (the orderly progression of pitch along the cochlea) of the array in the cochlear implant was terrible. The graph showed how the subject's perceived pitch changed with the position of the stimulation. Almost all the pitch change was between electrode 1 and 2. After that the pitch changed randomly. The best result was achieved at a stimulation rate of 50 pulses per second (pps); at

200 and 500 pps there was no tonotopic effect at all. Luckily things were not as bad as they looked, although no one had a good explanation for the problem.

Two research students under Dewhurst at the Department of Electrical Engineering at the UOM were trying to miniaturise the speech processor. They had started with a room full of equipment, trying to miniaturise each part. A box about the size of a television set was under construction. Seligman was supposed to help get it to work and Patrick was his boss. The box contained 12 large circuit boards. Seligman said that each of the boards worked some of the time, but he didn't remember them ever all working at the same time.

From the point of view of a complete outsider, it appeared that the way to go about the task was to make a clean start by looking at the objective and working out the simplest way of achieving it. In Seligman's spare time (rather, time stolen from the job he was employed to do) he decided to try it his way. At first it wasn't easy. He had to promise Patrick not to spend too much time on the new device and there were discussions about the wisdom of starting another speech processor before the first was completed. However, it wasn't too long before the simpler approach was demonstrated to be effective and from then on there was no looking back. A box the size of a binocular case was the prototype.

The speech-processing project now headed in the opposite direction, from a filterbank with simultaneous stimulation and channel interaction to extreme simplicity and economy of stimulation. Had the UOM team been successful with the filterbank approach, the technology of the day could have resulted in a large box of electronics and a further box of batteries. It is quite possible that they would never have received funding to go commercial with such a device. As it was, their somewhat impoverished strategy was relatively easy to implement in a box that could be worn on a belt or in a shirt pocket and which could run on a few AA cells.

Greg Cook, a technical officer, joined the UOM team after implantation of the first patient and some of the work of building the next two implants fell to Cook and Seligman. They were not concerned with any of the really tricky assembly but were involved in manufacture of the coils, which were a 'pancake' design backed by ferrite. The ferrite was taken from off-the-shelf potcores that were far too thick to be of use as they were. The team needed to thin them down. Previously the ferrite had been ground down by hand, using an old air-operated dentist's drill. The coils were wound between two Teflon spacers and potted in epoxy to hold the turns together. The coils were then fitted to the ferrite backplate and the whole assembly was coated with high-grade epoxy and baked in an oven.

Seligman tried to turn the ferrite on a lathe. Of course, the brittle material shattered. He then tried to put the handpiece of the dental drill into the tool-holder of the lathe and spin the diamond burr while slowly turning the chuck. In the end, he found that he could grind the ferrites very neatly on a machine called a surface grinder. The magnetic clutch held the ferrite very nicely.

Joe Tong was the UOM speech-processing and psychophysics guru whom Seligman asked about the new speech-coding strategy. Tong explained it in the time it took him and Seligman to cross Victoria Parade in Melbourne, a wide road opposite the hospital. Seligman took it from there.

The portable speech processor was a 'skunkworks' project, i.e. one that was not on the plan. But with support from Patrick, Seligman was able to work on it. At first it consisted of two 'breadboards' plugged into connectors on an aluminium frame. The rather fragile construction was wheeled about on a trolley. Saunders, the first implant recipient, came in week after week for testing. Frequently the poor man received loud 'bangs', which were mainly due to Seligman's fiddling with the power and data links. Eventually these issues were sorted out, and Cook and Seligman built a box of electronics that patients could carry around.

The portable speech processor did not drive the implant in the way it was intended to be driven. In the speech-coding strategy, the stimulation rate was the pitch of the speaker's voice. This was not something that was easily done with a fixed frame rate that the implant had been designed to implement. It would have required setting delay durations of each stimulus pulse to different numbers, something needing a lot of rapid calculation. To overcome this problem, Seligman used the implant in an unorthodox way. He simply stopped sending data until a glottal pulse (the puff of air through the speaker's larynx) was received, then sent the data without any adjustment. Thus the stimulation occurred in time with the speaker's voice pitch. He also tried sending power on demand, but that resulted in explosive sounds in the patient's head.

The results were promising and, given the success of the first implant, Clark pressed on to develop the concept further. To ensure access to government assistance, he wrote to the then prime minister, Malcolm Fraser. To build commercialisation capabilities, he wrote to both Trainor and the 3M company, asking for a meeting with whoever could provide the critical commercial backing. His efforts were rewarded and the Australian government, seeking to encourage high-tech development, became part of a necessary network in the project's development.

In the next two years, Clark and Trainor became close allies in driving the commercialisation of the cochlear implant project to fruition. The two men clearly respected each other which, given their similarities, is not surprising. Clark found that Trainor strove to ensure that the commercial effort dovetailed with the UOM research and, as time went on, they developed such a rapport in explaining their work at symposia that Trainor thought they performed like a 'Punch and Judy' show although Clark was never quite sure which one was Punch and which one was Judy.

CHAPTER 3

The champions in government: Ralph Tobias and Ian Macphee

'That'd be right,' he grumbled to himself. 'Thinks he's on a winner when all he's got are the crumbs. Wouldn't know a business opportunity if he fell over it.' Ralph Tobias angrily bundled his papers together and left yet another upsetting government department meeting in disgust.

In 1976 Tobias was first assistant secretary in the Department of Productivity, Science and Technology. He had graduated from university as an engineer and started public service life in 1952 in the Department of Civil Aviation, eventually moving through the Departments of Supply and Industry and Commerce. At that point he was responsible for the initiation and oversight of technology development projects aimed at developing Australian defence industry technology. The development included type-testing the final products for defence approval. But Tobias was more than that. He was a man on a mission. Over time he had noticed how technological ideas and initiatives that were developed in Australia were never bought by the Australian military. There was an apparent disjuncture between the ability to innovate and the ability to recognise the commercial value and possibilities of Australian research. The pervasive culture considered that something made in the USA or UK would obviously be superior to an Australian-designed and manufactured product. International networks had been established and international mateships often maintained the culture.

As the years progressed Tobias was able to influence some decisions to help the cause. On a visit to the Australian Research Laboratories in Adelaide, for instance, he learnt that the laboratories had been developing a sonobuoy system to detect submarines – the Nangana research project. This was exciting research and Tobias intuitively understood its possibilities. He asked what the researchers were going to do about it. Amused, they replied, 'We are not going to do anything about it. Our research work is done.' Tobias' eyes lit up and he asked if they had any objections to his following through with their research. Their work having been completed, they had no further interest and said, 'Sure, go for it.'

Putting his mission into operation, Tobias presented an initial introduction of the concept and a plan for how it could be taken through engineering development to a production system, to the Navy and Air Force headquarters. He then prepared the project plan and a funding submission to oversee commercial development of the technology. The concept was accepted and Tobias was given the role of Australian Program Director, in which he directed the creation of additional possibilities that expanded its use to airplanes. The additional development enabled him to begin negotiating the principles of a collaborative development with the UK. It was agreed that Australia would develop and produce the sonobuoys and the UK would develop and produce the airborne processor. Driven, Tobias negotiated the contracting arrangements to tap into the specialised capabilities of Australian firms CAC, AWA, Electronic Systems and Management Services (ESAMS) and Plessey. He simultaneously developed complex management arrangements involving the RAN, RAAF, WRE, UK Ministry of Defence and Australian and UK contractors. The development of the sonobuoy project was eventually transferred to the federal Department of Defence in 1976 and was ultimately completed to the original estimate of approximately $20 million. It was with some satisfaction that Tobias saw Australian production of the Barra sonobuoy ultimately earn more than $200 million from significant exports.

But after all that effort, when the RAAF wanted to replace its maritime patrol aircraft a few years later it chose to buy a US model. The UK model was available, as was a French plane. Tobias argued that the UK model would be a superior choice because it was already fitted with the Australian Barra system. Eventually recognising that he was not going to be successful in getting the RAAF to buy the UK model, Tobias proposed an engineering study to evaluate the feasibility of fitting the Barra airborne system to the US PC3 Orion, which normally came fitted with an inferior

US sonobuoy system. The study provided the basis for the project to install the Barra system in PC3s in Australia. The RAAF removed the US sonobuoy system and installed weapons systems that integrated the Barra system. The project also involved the design and construction of a local Barra training simulator, mission debrief and systems development facility. Although a long way from the best financial option, the project was at least completed by Australian companies and provided some positive outcomes for Australian technological innovation.

Similar episodes occurred, and Tobias' mission became a passion as he continued to see lost commercial opportunities for Australian technological inventions. Time and again he sat through yet another meeting, hearing applause for ridiculously low returns from licensing agreements instead of applause for what could have been a $1 billion Australian business.

It was not long before Tobias' passion was able to move to a new level of influence. In the mid 1970s the Whitlam Labor government was dismissed and the Liberal Party, with Malcolm Fraser as Prime Minister, came into power. By then Tobias was in the Department of Supply and he soon became part of the Department of Industry and Commerce. Opportunities soon presented themselves that would allow his white charger to go full speed ahead.

Tobias was requested by the Chairman of the Public Service Board, Sir Alan Cooley, to conduct an independent review of the public service-wide personnel and establishment system, Mandata, being developed by the board. He was excited by the challenge. He undertook the review and concluded that the project was in deep trouble, team morale was low, progress was very slow and the project was over-spending and over-ambitious. During the review process, Tobias involved the demoralised team in creating a solution to take the project forward. On presenting his report to the board he brought the team into the meeting to discuss the recommended solution for the project's troubles. The discussions led to collaborative solutions and brought a new enthusiasm into the project.

While Tobias was undertaking the Mandata review the Minister for Productivity, Ian Macphee, requested Sir Alan Cooley to become the new Secretary of the Department. Prime Minister Malcolm Fraser had created the Ministry for Productivity and appointed Ian Macphee to run it with the view of devising new policies to improve productivity created by paradigm shifts in the national economy. Throughout the 1970s, global economies were affected by two major events. The first was the development of the microchip, which revolutionised production processes and created increasing numbers of unemployed who were displaced by new technologies. Second was the announcement of oil price-fixing by the Organisation of Petroleum Exporting Countries (OPEC), which sent production prices and consequent inflation to frightening levels and established the need for greater efficiency in production processes. Early in November 1976, Ian Macphee was sworn in as Minister of Productivity, the most junior in the three industry departments – Industry and Commerce and Business and Consumer Affairs. He was charged with the task of developing policies that would prepare Australia for the inevitable and essential technology upheaval to come.

In his maiden speech Macphee stressed the importance of the three Ps – people, profit and productivity. 'Profit', he said, 'should not be a dirty word to unions and people should not be a dirty word to management. On the contrary, they are the principal asset. Industrial democracy is the key where unions and management can work together for a similar objective and at least have a defined goal instead of always being confrontational.' He was an early advocate of moving personnel officers out of the back corridor into the board room and changing their titles from personnel officers to human resource directors. He insisted that people were a resource to be invested in, not a cost to be contained. On being sworn into his portfolio, Macphee focused on job redesign and promoted the benefit of computer technology although at the time a computer filled three small bedrooms. He stressed the importance of computers in design and manufacture and championed the connection between job security, job rotation, multi-skilling and productivity.

But Macphee was a minority voice in the Fraser government. In the late 1970s the Liberal Party included the 'new right', who were followers of the economic theories espoused by Milton Friedman and known as 'economic rationalism'. Within the party, economic rationalists were known more familiarly as the 'dries'. On either side of the House, anyone wanting to prioritise social development or welfare measures was dubbed 'wet' and, by implication, irrational. To conservative parties in the UK, Europe and the USA as well as Australia, economic rationalism was attractive as a coherent reworking of the classic laissez-faire economics at the source of 18th-century liberalism. Proponents within the Fraser government were Australia's equivalent of the Thatcherites in Britain and the Reaganites in the USA.

This was not an easy environment in which the most junior minister in Cabinet could garner empathy for industrial democracy. Such sentiments put Macphee firmly in the 'wet' camp. But despite the dismissal of his ideas by the dries, who included Treasury, he relentlessly argued for the creation of new industries such as biotechnology. He emphasised that 'an essential element of a healthy private sector is important in maintaining an aggressive, competitive outlook by business leaders, but it is competition from new products, new processes and new organisations that injects real stimulus to a successful, expanding and prosperous manufacturing industry'. It was with the objective of improving national competitiveness that a Public Interest Grant was established.

Late one evening, sitting in his office while the shadows outside blended into darkness, Tobias responded to a knock on the door which was followed by an invitation to go to the local bar. Over a friendly ale, the details of Macphee's search for interesting projects were related and he was asked if he could create a taskforce to figure out how the department could go about finding appropriate projects. Would he be interested in heading the project? Tobias saw the door of opportunity open, and accepted the assignment with enthusiasm.

His acceptance of the challenge was a little hasty, however. He was still running the Department of Industry and Commerce and taking on the position of First Assistant Secretary in the Departments of Productivity and Science and Technology meant that for about eight months he was in the tricky position of having responsibility for two departments. But Tobias loved it. This was what he had been working towards for at least 20 years. With the thrill of anticipated success he started looking at what could be done to make up for the previous loss of opportunities. It was obvious that the Minister's dilemma revolved around the fact that although the IR&D legislation in 1977 provided provision for 'public interest projects', none had been identified to that date. Seeing the opportunity for an innovative way of supporting the commercial development of Australian invention and technology, funds had been sought and secured to support such projects. But, since none had been undertaken, procedures and processes had to be formulated from scratch. This was done immediately, and a number of projects were identified and evaluated.

The rationale behind the public interest program depended on a simple equation that demonstrated the need for government assistance for companies that wished to commercialise worthwhile Australian innovations but whose management was unable to make the investment in R&D necessary to take that innovation to market.

To place this in perspective, the average industry spend on R&D at that time was substantially less than 2% of sales. If a company had an R&D project which would require an R&D expenditure of $1 million a year, it would be highly unlikely to allocate its entire R&D budget to that one project. Prudent managers would want to spread their R&D investment risk over several projects. If the company decided to spend a quarter of its R&D budget on the one project, this would mean that the company's R&D budget would need to be $4 million a year. If the R&D budget were 2% of sales (a figure above the industry average) then the company would need sales of at least $200 million per year. This ratio would scale up with larger project R&D expenditures. Proportionately higher project R&D expenditures would require companies with proportionally higher sales figures. In some product areas, Australia had few if any such companies.

This thinking led to the Department of Productivity view that there were worthwhile Australian R&D projects that would never happen without external financial input, or at least would not happen in Australia. The Australian investment community had little interest in providing external financial input to research projects, leading to the inevitable losses to Australian competitiveness, to potential export earnings, to local employment and to the growth of related industries desperately needed in the Australian economy to combat rising unemployment. To reverse the trend of declining international competitiveness in Australian industry, Macphee recognised that his department had to adopt a leading role by undertaking, with the assistance of industry, major R&D projects.

The first project was with ICI. ICI had a licence from CSIRO technology for purifying water but was having great difficulty in getting the project off the ground because the public authorities would need to build large water purification plants to prove the technology. Until it was proven it couldn't be sold, but the financial investment and therefore the risk in obtaining the proof was substantial. The first public interest project thus involved building a water purification plant in Perth, Western Australia, with the water authorities. The aim was to provide proof of concept so that technology could be commercialised. The project succeeded.

One of the early public interest projects brought to Tobias' attention was the bionic ear proposal from Professor Graeme Clark at the University of Melbourne (UOM). One day a staff member came into Tobias' office, announcing that he had found an excellent public benefit project. He said it was a beauty. A bionic ear sounded pretty inspiring to the entrepreneurial engineer. 'Unfortunately', said the staffer, 'there is good and bad news about it.' The bad news was that the UOM had given away the first option on the bionic ear technology to 3M, a US company, so the innovation might be lost to Australia. 'What is the good news?' Tobias asked. The good news was that the option expired in three months.

Crucially, the bionic ear was a perfect fit to the department's policy objectives of nurturing a high-technology base and countering the trend of Australian innovations being lost to foreign companies. Tobias flew to Melbourne to meet Clark. 'Would you like us to do something to help you commercialise this work?' asked Tobias. Clark was ecstatic, but impatient that they still had to wait for three months to see what 3M would do. Nothing happened. 3M decided that it would back the rival US single-electrode device being developed by Bill House and the House Institute. 3M's decision to move away from the UOM device allowed the Department of Productivity to take steps to provide the bridge between research and industry.

The project greatly stimulated Macphee's interest. The hearing-impaired had long been a concern for him. He had been in kindergarten with a little girl who had a serious hearing defect and, although he had been amazed to see how well she managed, it was exciting to know that there was an innovation that might assist people like her. Consequently, when Macphee learnt of the painstaking research and the need for more research he supported the project enthusiastically, especially after meeting Clark himself.

Although he had great respect for Departmental Secretaries Alan Cooley and Ralph Tobias, Macphee could not just depend on what they said. He needed to double-check the details to fill the gaps in his own knowledge so that he would be fully prepared when arguing in Cabinet for funding. He had to be especially sure about the facts in this case since he was promoting a bionic ear which, at the time, sounded more like a television program than serious research. The dries argued that it was a private sector issue and if it was worth doing it should be done by industry not by government. Wasting taxpayers' money on something that sounded like science fiction was something that they could not condone. Macphee did not give up.

By this time two Nucleus subsidiaries, Telectronics and Ausonics, had established reputations for innovation and research and had gained international recognition in biomedical engineering and market acceptance, in terms of heart pacemakers and diagnostic ultrasound. Telectronics had established manufacturing and marketing subsidiaries worldwide and Ausonics was launching the first water-path-based diagnostic ultrasound scanning system for obstetrics and cardiology. Paul Trainor and his Nucleus Group were becoming well known in the medical devices community.

Macphee was not particularly concerned about formality. He needed to get to the bottom of the bionic ear proposal and wasn't going to wait for official advice. He called Trainor to gauge his interest. Trainor asked for two weeks, during which time he made international phone calls to determine what research had already been done and what industrialisation had been achieved in the area. He received sufficient information to warrant sending a small team to the UOM to investigate the viability of the cochlear implant and the feasibility of the technology. Trainor had a competent team of technical, legal and commercial experts which had reviewed over 300 such projects in various multi-disciplinary research fields. The initial response was always 'Let's explore it more carefully', but on this occasion it appeared that there was real potential.

Given this advice, Macphee was able to argue that recipients of the device would gain enormous benefit whether they lived in Australia or not. It was something that the government was morally obliged to do. Australia had the sciences to achieve this goal but it required taxpayers' support. On hearing that Treasury was advising rejection of his request for IR&D funding for the bionic ear, Macphee went privately to Prime Minister Malcolm Fraser for support – and got it. With additional and crucial strong support from highly respected and influential colleagues, Doug Anthony and Peter Nixon, National Party members of the Coalition, Macphee managed to push through approval for a $400 000 grant. No one in Cabinet had any doubt after he had presented the argument that if it were successful there would be more requests to take the prototype to commercial success.

The department called a meeting of interested parties in Canberra late in 1978. At the meeting the department indicated that it was prepared to award Clark a public interest grant that would fund the next phase of development, which it was agreed would consist of two steps. The first step focused on ensuring that the scheme really worked. The second step required market and cost analyses to be undertaken to determine if there were sufficient worldwide demand, before a final decision was made to proceed with development. It was considered necessary that, to give some confidence to the project, an international market survey and cost estimates should be completed within a nine-month period. It was agreed that if these conditions were met, the government would provide the risk capital for development of the device subject to it being commercialised in Australia. This was to be followed by the implantation of six more patients with a fully re-engineered system.

Macphee announced the $400 000 public interest grant on 31 January 1979, and the following day advertised for expressions of interest from companies willing to undertake a market survey and development cost plan. Telectronics was one of seven companies invited to bid and one of only two which submitted a tender. The Telectronics tender highlighted the company's track record and considerable experience in the development and marketing of implantable electronic devices: 'We feel we are admirably suited to carry out this project as it is of a generally similar nature to the work which we have to do for any introduction of new products of our own.'

The Department of Productivity concurred with these claims in its evaluation of the Telectronics bid. The company had in-house R&D and manufacturing capabilities for implantable devices, which meant that the development cost plan would be conducted by people who were aware of the manufacturing challenges likely to be encountered. The company's marketing expertise was also appropriate. Telectronics had recently completed a similar marketing plan for its latest invention, the bone growth stimulator. The cochlear implant was a medical implant whose commercialisation would, like that of pacemakers, require depth of experience in technology, medical regulatory disciplines and approvals on a global scale, plus the manufacturing and marketing skills that would ensure acceptance. Telectronics also thoroughly understood the financial planning of such a project. The company knew from previous experience that the project would take 10 years from prototype to accepted medically approved (FDA) implant. Concurrently with R&D on the implant there would have to be clinical trials, documentation, payment of fees to audiologists worldwide, back-up clinical research and submissions to the FDA – no one had done such a project before, especially on a global scale. The company's early assessment was that the R&D/clinical trials/pre-market FDA approval trials/documentation/good manufacturing practice would cost (in 1980 terms) around $A10 million per year. As Trainor later summed it up, Telectronics was the logical choice and arguably the only company in Australia at the time with the required industrial and international experience. It therefore was the logical choice to win the government contract, and commenced work in July 1979.

In the first phase a steering committee was set up by the Australian Industrial Research and Development Incentives Board (AIR&DIB), chaired by an Assistant Secretary of the Department of Productivity. The UOM team and Telectronics were part of the committee and reported on their progress. The UOM implanted two more subjects while Telectronics conducted a market survey and prepared a development cost plan. Their final reports were submitted in December 1979, and based on them the department decided to recommend a second phase of funding.

In Phase 2, $1.5 million was granted for the design and construction of a prototype clinical system that would be fitted to six volunteers during Phase 3, in late 1982. Telectronics began making the hardware improvements that would make the prototype a commercially manufacturable product. Nucleus itself now became the contractual party, rather than its subsidiary Telectronics. Telectronics' management and its French shareholder, the pharmaceutical company Synthelabo, considered that the cochlear implant project did not fit with the company's plans and the potential return on investment was seen as being too far in the future so they consented to the project's move into the Nucleus Group.

The government did not guarantee funding beyond each phase. In 1982, at the end of Phase 2 when the implant was ready to undergo clinical trials, Nucleus made a submission to the Department of Productivity (reorganised and renamed the Department of Science and Technology), requesting that government funding be continued because 'at this stage in Nucleus' growth it is not possible to fund such a high-risk project'. Nucleus was under additional pressure, having suffered a loss in 1982 due to problems with the development of a second-generation diagnostic ultrasound. The Nucleus report stressed the long lead times before medical products become profitable, and the fact that the implant was yet to receive regulatory approval. An independent consultant commissioned by the government agreed with Nucleus' assessment of the degree of risk. The Department of Science and Technology agreed that it would fund 75% of Phase 3, with Nucleus contributing the remainder.

Phase 3 of government funding was publicly announced in late 1982. It differed from earlier rounds in that not only was it the largest (at $2.3 million), but it was the first time in which more funding was going to Nucleus as the commercial partner rather than to the basic research being conducted by the UOM team. In a contract signed with a government agency, Nucleus committed to delivering a prosthesis that was ready for clinical trials. Conditional upon this agreement was the negotiation of an exclusive worldwide agreement between Nucleus as licensee, and the government and UOM as joint licensors. The licensing agreement, signed in December 1982, provided the licensors with a joint share of royalties amounting to 5% of sales of the first 12 000 units and 2% thereafter. Nucleus won the right to sublicense, although any move to manufacture offshore would require approval from the licensors.

In total, four rounds of government funding took place from 1979–85, totalling about $4.7 million. Although it was not prepared to fund the full cost of clinical trials for the cochlear implant, Nucleus' submission had emphasised that the company would be ready to assume responsibility for commercialisation at the end of Phase 4. 'This project is particularly important to Nucleus Ltd because of its potential for diversification within the high-technology health care field,' Trainor explained. The cochlear project was a very good fit for the company's strategy, which was to innovate and develop products which as much as possible represented an advance in applied technology rather than merely duplicated products that already existed in the market.

However, despite government contributions for seed and early-stage development, in 1983 the company was still several years from the projected cashflow break-even point, which was not expected until 1986. Trainor was unwilling to bear the burden of funding for that entire period. Cochlear Pty Ltd was established in 1983 partly to facilitate external fundraising. The revised estimate was that an additional $5 million was required to take the company through to cashflow break-even, and Trainor was determined that at least $3 million of it would have to be raised from external sources.

Until the mid 1980s the Australian financing community had been subject to a tightly regulated financial system and it was very conservative and inexperienced in sophisticated financial markets. It was particularly risk-averse with respect to technology-based investing. There were few venture capital investors, and very few precedents that investors could use to determine approximate value of the company and the risks involved in Australian companies that planned to dominate global markets with novel technologies. The federal government's management investment company (MIC) program was initiated to promote the development of a venture capital industry in Australia as a means of fostering Australian technology-based companies. Fortuitously, this initiative created a new pool of possible investment funds for Cochlear Pty Ltd.

One of the challenges facing the new company was the fact that none of the funding so far had been in the form of an equity investment. There was no previous round of funding to refer to. A net present value of projected cashflows was calculated by David Money and verified by Price Waterhouse, yielding a value of $20 million. Trainor understood that overseas, particularly in the USA, venture capital industries were experienced in best-quality science, particularly in the biotechnology sector. Trainor knew that, to establish a real value for the fledgling company, it would be necessary to go outside the Australian financial community. He was also determined that Cochlear Pty Ltd would only accept Australian financing if the financial terms were almost as good as those that he could establish with players from the global market. However, the availability of further government grants and other non-dilutive government funding would become an issue if ownership of the company went offshore.

In the second half of 1983, Bear Sterns New York was retained to help Trainor identify international venture capital investors for $3 million first-round financing. He selected a New York-based merchant bank, to give the small Australian company the credibility which would be critical in discussions with experienced finance groups in Europe and the USA.

The timing was excellent. In the USA there had been a revolution in the approach to the commercialisation of medical research. The biotech revolution had begun and venture capitalists carried the entrepreneurial spirit generated in Silicon Valley in the 1960s and 1970s into the biotech spinoffs from university research labs. The biotech world really changed on 14 October 1980, when Blyth Eastman Paine Webber and San Francisco boutique bank Hambrecht & Quist took Genentech Inc., the first biotech company to be listed on the stock exchange, public. The extraordinary positive response to the listing provided an impetus to firms like Cochlear. Within a few months Trainor's team had secured an offer of $A3 million to buy 27.5% of the equity in Cochlear Corp., a US-based company that would own the rights to Cochlear Pty Ltd's technology, from Fred Adler. Adler was renowned for successful venture capital investments in the computer industry.

The offer, by an international player with expertise in high-technology investment, set a value for Cochlear Pty Ltd. Accepting this investment had several attractive features. It was a firm offer from an investor that was US-based and could do much to support the establishment of US operations and to smooth the US regulatory process. If the planned exit from the investment was a NASDAQ listing, the support of US-based venture capital investors would be very valuable. The price recognised a significant improvement on the funds attracted to date, a factor that would satisfy Nucleus Ltd and the federal government alike. However, surrendering significant ownership of the company to a non-Australian partner would not be attractive to the government.

In addition to the international fundraising effort, Trainor courted Australian investors. By mid 1984 three independent venture capital groups, two with funds raised under the MIC scheme, had expressed interest in investing small amounts in Cochlear Pty Ltd. Trainor preferred a syndicated investment, which was offered by Nick Callinan of Western Pacific in Melbourne.

Western Pacific had raised a $10 million fund in May 1984 under the MIC scheme, providing investors in the government-licensed fund with a 100% tax deduction for the capital they had committed to the fund on condition that they maintained their investment for a minimum of four years. This was enough time to take Cochlear to break-even point. The MIC fund was constrained to invest only in early-stage, technology-based Australian companies with a strong export orientation – exactly Cochlear's position.

In late 1984 the Australian syndicate Western Pacific made an offer to buy 27.5% of Cochlear Pty Ltd for $3 million. Trainor therefore had a choice of two offers, and the Australian offer made greater sense. Cochlear Pty Ltd would remain Australian operated and owned and would have the support of local venture capital with a strongly commercial approach. This was clearly important to the Australian staff, to the Australian government which had provided the early-stage funding and to the Australian management team. Control of the company and the location of manufacturing and other operations would be linked to the nationality of the investor group. The Australian syndicate of investors also provided some capacity for future financing, if this was necessary due to longer than anticipated clinical trials or other regulatory procedures. Therefore the market was not surprised to hear that the Cochlear board decided to choose the locally based investor over the US-based offer. The offer was acceptable to the Australian government and Trainor became confident that the development could proceed at least to break-even point.

In his book *Sounds from Silence*, Clark acknowledged the outstanding way in which the 'bureaucrats' handled the project. He thanked Paul Schultz, Frank Montgomery, Geoff Tunaley, Nick Sterling and Ted Cowcher. David Money also acknowledged the efforts of the steering committee and commented that, as well as providing vital funding, the committee was useful in managing the relationship between UOM and the company, encouraging an additional discipline in both.

It is often said that the biotechnology industry eventuated through a triple helix of government, industry and academia. In the USA this liaison operates very effectively and it is not surprising that the USA is the industry leader by many multiples. For each technology, a champion from each of the three sectors is a prerequisite. If such an industry is to flourish in Australia there has to be government assistance right from the start and there have to be champions in the government who will kick it off and keep it going. Without these ingredients, it is difficult to see how the industry can prosper in a small country such as Australia. Trainor always acknowledged that Cochlear Pty Ltd was the outcome of a three-way partnership of university, government and industry. It had not one but three organisations involved in its founding: the Department of Productivity, the UOM and the Nucleus Group.

CHAPTER 4

Engineers were vital: David Money and others

The autumn rain flicked from its destination by the windscreen wipers' hypnotic rhythm gently trickled down the window frame as David Money urged his car home to his young family. It was late but they were used to seeing him arrive well after dark. He and his colleagues worked long hours but it was a labour of love, and tonight Money had an additional air of satisfaction.

In his school days Money could not decide if he were going to be a doctor, a lawyer or an engineer. In the end he chose electrical engineering at a time when the industry was on the cusp of a revolutionary era. He managed to secure a job with AWA and became involved in setting up the integrated circuit industry in Australia. At the time, as in all paradigm shifts, some doubted the industry's ability to survive. But survive it did, and Money was among those leading the charge as an integrated circuit designer. In the 1960s he designed a wide variety of circuits including hearing aids and pacemakers, and rose to the role of general manager of research and development. In that role he succeeded in convincing Paul Trainor's Telectronics that the only way to obtain sufficient reliability in pacemakers was to use AWA integrated circuits designed by him.

His years at AWA were interesting but after a particularly intense June when Trainor had ramped up pressure on the small engineering company by increasing production demand for Telectronics integrated circuits, doubling and then tripling production – creating what became known as the red-eye project – the researcher in Money wondered why on earth he had given up the lab bench for management. To make his life even more difficult, Telectronics cut its requirement to a minimum once the new financial year began. This strategy helped Telectronics appease the Australian Taxation Office but, for the general manager of a small production company, the vacillation in production demand created a stress level that was not worth the effort. After 15 years Money needed a change. Telectronics heard of his search for a change; it was delighted and welcomed him with open arms in 1969. It offered him an interesting series of roles including production engineering, manufacturing, and setting up quality assurance processes. He eventually became Head of Applied Research when Geoffrey Wickham retired from that role. It was then that Money had his first contact with the University of Melbourne (UOM) team and their bionic ear prototype.

Sitting in his office at the top of the stairs, next to Trainor's office in the Nucleus premises at Lane Cove in Sydney, Money contemplated the UOM device. Budgets were very tight at Telectronics so he was somewhere between outraged and shocked to learn that Wickham had agreed to pay $400 just to look at a collection of patents from the UOM. Money was acutely aware of the enormous distance between a prototype manufactured by a university and the creation of a marketable product that could be commercially successful. A prototype was designed to last a few years, to test whether the concept worked. The obvious next step would be for the UOM to contact a group that had the technological expertise to commercialise it. Why, he angrily wondered, was it necessary to pay for patents when the UOM should have been begging Nucleus to take on the commercialisation process? The patents did, however, indicate that the research could provide a variety of different avenues for Telectronics and Money proceeded to investigate its commercial development.

Wickham, as a director of Telectronics and a friend of David Dewhurst from the UOM, had recommended to the Nucleus Group board that the project be taken on but Trainor and Money needed a lot more convincing. Money thought that the project was an extraordinarily impressive design for a university to have carried through to prototype. Although he was impressed by the technological advance that the cochlear prosthesis represented, he was convinced that it would fail if implanted in a human. His assessment was that the device was a beautiful work of art but a complete redesign would be necessary for it to be made more reliable.

To develop the new design, Money worked with one of the best and most experienced electronic designers from Telectronics, Chris Daly. Together they flew to Melbourne to see for themselves exactly what the UOM had achieved. On the flight back to Sydney, they brainstormed an entirely different system. Returning to Telectronics, they devised a radically simplified design that represented a considerable inventive step. The original prototype had almost 50 integrated circuit chips, two coils (one for the provision of power and the other for data) and a speech processor that had to be connected to a minicomputer for the essential programming of individual patients. The new design contained a single integrated circuit, one coil for both power and data, and it envisaged a diagnostic and programming unit that could be controlled by a home computer. The new design would deliver not only improved reliability but greater capability as well. It would also be able to stimulate 22 sites in the inner ear rather than the 10 sites stimulated by the prototype. Their broad-brush functional design seemed to satisfy all the basic requirements for commercial development. Money smiled as he drove home, knowing they had taken the first step to overcoming a potential barrier to commercial development. That afternoon, with the assistance of Nucleus' very smart patent lawyer, Mike Rackman, they had initiated a patent application for the new design. Sitting in the dark car with the sound of the windscreen wipers and the gentle thud of the rain, it was satisfying to know that Telectronics was in a position to use the commercial design as the basis for a cost plan on which subsequent development work could be based.

Money had been involved in the initial discussions with the federal government and had feared that this was too big a deal for Nucleus, because of its very high risk and its obviously very high investment requirement. That level of risk-taking was pretty extraordinary and not what would be expected from a company like Nucleus. His thoughts were not well received and Money didn't want to just say no – there might, after all, be possibilities in the project. But he was certain that they couldn't just say yes, because of the large amount of risk. The Nucleus Group needed time to find out what it would actually be in for. Money was therefore relieved that Trainor declined the initial offer from the government and insisted that a market study be done first. That had given them time to investigate the possibilities before any commitment was made. There were so many areas where major revisions to the approach were needed and these had to be defined before any development could be carried out. Nucleus needed to have some sort of idea what it was dealing with and had to have the concept in mind; it even had to know how big a project development of the cochlear implant was going to be. The early design implant was not manageable from a manufacturing point of view. The coding scheme, dual transmission, sealing technology – it all added up to a very complicated, very sophisticated system. That is not how to make something reliable.

The ultimate tenderer would need to know what it was in for so the government asked for tenders in stages, with a market survey as part of the first stage. This strategy meant, however, that the idea had to be developed and the patent applied for when Nucleus/Telectronics was not receiving government funding. The company was only taking an interest in becoming involved and it could easily have ended up as a very expensive experiment. But, with the patent lodged, Money knew they had achieved a critical step. He was also confident that the Daly/Money patent would be important in negotiations with the government over why the contract should be awarded to the Australian company, if the market study indicated the need for development of the prototype. It did indeed turn out to be useful in winning the tender, because the patent seemed to have a number of key points which were an improvement on anything else in the field and it gave Telectronics an edge over other tenderers. But Ralph Tobias drew Money's attention to the fact that a piece of wartime legislation, still current, enabled the Australian government to assume all rights to all Australian inventions without having to make payment. The weapon Money was counting on was not as safe as he thought, but the comfort was that the design was still the best available.

Now that Telectronics/Nucleus had patented the design it was able to develop a reliable cost plan which could include the cost of actually doing the design, getting prototypes of the integrated circuits and the manufacturing cost of the forecast volumes. The plan would also enable Telectronics, under the umbrella of Nucleus, to submit a well-researched tender for the government grant being offered to manufacture the cochlear implant.

Money had no idea how many people could benefit from such a device and he was certain that neither did anyone else. There were statistics on the number of people using a hearing aid but a device for the profoundly deaf was another matter, and estimating the demand was another barrier that could derail the project. It was critical that a rough estimate be made because experience had taught the Nucleus Group that the commercialisation process was long and very expensive. Without sufficient demand there was no use in even beginning the project. Money wondered whether the new patent would be any use after all.

The market study was going to be the deciding factor and Money had finally managed to convince Jim Loughman, head of Telectronics International Marketing, to provide resources to undertake such a study.

CHAPTER 5

A marketeer and a doctor provide evidence of demand: the market study

'I'm not doing it!' she shouted, her voice echoing over the functional wood partitions in the low-key unpretentious office that separated them from the rest of the Telectronics staff in their equally basic workspaces. Before coming to Australia Maria Yetton had worked in market research in the UK and the USA. She was the first woman in the UK to be awarded an MBA, way back in 1967. When she came to Australia in 1976 she had made up her mind that she was going into senior line management. She couldn't have chosen a worse time or place to make such a career decision, but the decision had been made and she moved quickly up the corporate ladder. After a couple of job switches, she eventually joined Telectronics in 1978, employed by Jim Loughman. It was not an easy start, with Paul Trainor walking in and out of the interview saying, 'You know that I don't agree with this appointment.'

Despite Trainor's disapproval, Yetton got the job. Loughman was older than her and treated her like a clever but naughty daughter. Colleagues at Telectronics were used to hearing the two arguing. They were always fighting. He would shout at her, often using very colourful language, and she always shouted back. It was an odd relationship but it worked. There was respect on each side and the arguments were about professional issues, never personal. It was that kind of culture in the whole of the Nucleus organisation under Trainor. When Trainor decided to restructure the organisation, making Loughman CEO of the Nucleus Group, Loughman promoted Yetton to his job. Just months before the Cochlear tender, Yetton had secured a job that she thought was worthy of her – head of international marketing in a company that was recognised as a leader in the world of pacemakers. She was responsible for the marketing in 49 countries and for a really big team of employees. The job involved time away from home at international conferences, supporting 'their' doctors and displaying Telectronics products, networking and entertaining. With all this at her fingertips, Loughman told Yetton that she had to do a market survey for Cochlear. She didn't want to do the market survey. She had the job she wanted. She wanted to start getting to grips with that new job, not run around the globe gathering data for some implant that in all likelihood had absolutely no future.

Loughman was having none of it. The organisation had always been run like a family company, with Trainor the obvious man in charge. Loughman was similarly paternalistic. There was no arguing with his decisions. Employees were going to do what he wanted because he said so. He liked Yetton and wanted her to succeed. She had spirit and was not easily intimidated. He also knew that she was the best person to undertake a market study that would determine if there was enough demand for an invention that was supposed to make deaf people hear. Her skills had been demonstrated long before coming to Telectronics, during her work in a market research agency in the USA which specialised in new product forecasting. The work had focused on analysing new product launches and trials. Using that information to forecast whether the product was going to be a success or a dud, and the expected speed of product take-up, was always a challenging task.

Loughman knew that the marketing project he was giving Yetton was in her blood. She understood how to look at the initial sales curve to determine quickly if the product was going to take off. This was the sort of critical skill needed to put together a credible business plan that would convince the government to provide the substantial funding needed to make the project work, and give a national return. Or the data provided by the survey might suggest that it was in everyone's interest to walk away from the project. Even more importantly, from Loughman's point of view, the successful tender for the market research survey had specified the application of Yetton's experience and skills, a key factor of which she was completely unaware.

'You are the only person in this company that can do it. You have to do it', he repeated. There were two options open to Yetton. The first was to walk away from the company, which she was not prepared to do. The second was to accept the task and put the real job on hold for a while. She was well aware that senior management in Nucleus/Telectronics was extremely autocratic – Trainor and Loughman decided what would be done and who would do it. They allocated the jobs and Yetton had seen quite a few people who, despite kicking and screaming, were nevertheless forced to begin a task. Paramount to the success of this type of management was the fact that once the reluctant employee had calmed down and accepted their fate, they were very much left to get on with the task and do it their own way. Ultimately, therefore, jobs became rewarding, with great autonomy and hence satisfaction and typically they were done well. Because the company only recruited people who had significant talent and were also pretty individualistic, this style of management by creative tension worked despite creating a lot of stress and being highly unusual.

Yetton responded in the only way she could. 'Well, if I have to do it then I am going do it exactly how I want to. I will have exactly the scope and the type of people that I want involved. What's more, if I come back and I don't believe that this is the way to go then I am not going to be influenced by anyone. I am going to make a recommendation based on the data. I will tell it like it is.' Loughman had no problem with any of that. He just said, 'Okay, you just go and do it. We have $100 000 for the project, so go and do a first-class piece of research. You know what to do and I am not going to tell you what or how to do it, but in the meantime why not go to Melbourne and have a look at what they're doing? We need a report in six months.' Defiant in defeat, Yetton walked out the door, already focusing on the problems that would dominate her life for the next six months.

Previous experience had taught her that it would be a huge problem to define. What is the market size for something for which there is no real evidence that it will even work? There was no way of knowing who the device would suit. Yetton would have to determine which markets would be able to afford it, and where there were enough skilled surgeons and rehabilitation experts. More importantly, was anyone interested in undertaking the necessary training and investment? The first step was to split the various issues of demand. Which countries could provide a market? Which patients were the best to implant? What auditory conditions were required before an implant could take place? The levels of research would need to go from the general to the specific. There was also the question of potential market trail-off. The number of profoundly deaf people appeared to decline as medical standards improved. What would happen when the current market ran out? The future market appeared to be quite small, and declining. Could children be implanted? The task presented an enormous challenge but it did begin to stimulate Yetton's intellectual curiosity.

Telectronics, as one of the largest global companies in biocompatible implantable devices, had a wealth of experience and knowhow about such devices. Telectronics dominated the pacemaker market in Australia and was a major player in the USA, UK, France and many other countries. In essence, it was an upside-down multinational and for a long time had been providing resources, knowledge and even parking spaces around the world for the Nucleus Group and its people. There was always someone who could be contacted to do the local legwork and provide vital background information. David Money, head of R&D for Telectronics, did not appear to have any major concerns about the engineering obstacles to commercialisation of the cochlear implant. Yetton respected him a great deal and considered him to be a brilliant engineer. Had Money been concerned, Yetton would have been worried. She, like most others in the company, had absolute confidence in Money and his capabilities. If he thought commercialisation was possible, then it probably was. If he wasn't fazed there had to be a fighting chance that it was do-able.

The Nucleus Group understood that the international marketing of medical devices involved looking at each country and its medical system and its patients, individually. As well as looking at doctors and hospitals, it had to explore which countries had medical system insurance or government support funding for a device. The range was from the USA, where insurance was available to cover just about everything, to India where the patient had to pay for everything themselves. The company would need to explore the contrasts and look at the economics. It had no idea how the implant would work outside the English-speaking world. How would the implant cope with different tonal variations within language? Chinese, for instance, had very different tonal issues from Italian or English. Would the implant work in a non-English speaking context?

Since the Nucleus Group was looking at a start-up situation it would be important to consider the enabling factors such as the health regulation system, healthcare funding and, significantly, where to get good statistics. The next level of research would focus on the location of surgeons who would be capable of doing the implant.

Yetton began to develop a decision tree which would result in an estimate of the market size.

In 1978 Mike Hirshorn was a young man in his 20s. He had studied to be a doctor: when he thought about why he had chosen that path, he realised that perhaps it was due mainly to family expectation rather than to his own preference. He enjoyed the pursuit of his medical degree but when he had graduated and it came to looking after patients, it was not for him. Leaving Melbourne, he enrolled in an MBA course in Sydney and convinced Trainor to employ him. He was determined to demonstrate to his family and friends in Melbourne that his perceived step down from a medical career into the dubious world of trade was in fact a positive move. Involvement in such important research as the cochlear implant market study was, after all, what he was trained for. His medical skills made him the obvious person to talk to the medical researchers who would be encountered during the market study, and his MBA allowed him to understand the business requirements of such a venture. Hirshorn felt that he should have been given the job of leading the research.

Yetton was content for Hirshorn to work on certain aspects of the project, but not to assume overall leadership. She hadn't wanted to take on the project in the first place but, having grudgingly accepted it, she made it clear that it was she who decided who did what on the project. Hirshorn challenged her position, demanding that they discuss it with Loughman. That was fine with Yetton. She knew Loughman well enough to know what he would say. Together they marched into Loughman's office and Hirshorn demanded that Yetton be made aware that his qualifications meant that he should be boss of the market survey. He was stunned when Loughman disagreed and said, 'No, she's the boss.' This was not a good start to a project that demanded close contact and collaboration during a two-month overseas fact-finding trip. But, as always in the organisation, once the fighting was over they got on with doing a first-class job.

Having determined the structure and respective roles of the interviewing team, Yetton and Hirshorn went to Melbourne to see what the fuss was all about. Yetton's first impression of the cochlear implant was a room full of electronic equipment and boxes from floor to ceiling. The patient looked very small in comparison. The engineering challenge was clearly staggering. The huge amount of equipment would all have to be miniaturised to create a transportable and wearable device, and Yetton doubted whether it would ever be possible. But she was not at all technical and the engineers, though acknowledging the size of the challenge, were not unduly daunted.

Shrugging her shoulders, Yetton thought, 'Okay. I will go and evaluate the concept because I have been told to but at this point I don't believe in it and I think its chances are slim.' Little did she realise the convert that she would become – and converts often make the best advocates.

In its very broadest terms, the market survey she and Hirshorn worked on was designed to establish, on a worldwide basis:

- the total size of the available market and the subdivision of that market in terms of major marketing regions such as the USA, Europe, the eastern bloc, the Middle East and Asia;

- the existence of any market constraints such as acceptability criteria for implants imposed by regulatory bodies such as the US FDA or other regional health organisations and potential inhibitors to market acceptance among practitioners;

- the extent of potential competition from other commercial or research interests working in the field.

Yetton knew that it was necessary to refine each of those broad objectives into a number of much more specific objectives. In developing those objectives she created the agenda for an overseas trip to assess the market, along with the necessary statistical and economic research elements that could be done from Australia. First and foremost were the questions of market size and market constraints. Market size is a somewhat loosely used phrase in this instance, since estimates can be made at a number of different levels. Three prime levels were identified and research programs were designed and conducted at each level.

The first was the ultimate consumer or patient level. At this level, the major requirement was to identify the total number of profoundly deaf people in each of the identified geographic market areas. It was then necessary to identify the essential demographics of the profoundly deaf such as age, sex, economic and social status. There were also specific market segments for individual attention, such as the numbers of pre-lingually and post-lingually deaf, in order to determine the market potential of each segment, as their communication needs would vary.

There were potential constraints on market size at this level, such as the degree to which demographic factors such as age might reduce the total available market, for instance, the appropriateness of the implant for young children. Conversely, how appropriate would the device be for older patients in whom both the process of learning and current experience levels would be totally dissimilar from those of the average adult population? This was a critical issue. Psychological factors, including emotional and cognitive learning factors, also had to be considered. Such factors would all affect, and potentially reduce, the total number of patients for whom the implant would be appropriate.

A second factor which was critical in assessing market size was the number of appropriate hospitals or implanting locations. It was necessary to collect data on the number of available hospitals or locations within each market area that had the staff and resource capacity to implant an electronic prosthetic hearing device, not only current ones but also those likely to be available within the next five years. Ideally, this would entail an investigation of broad parameters such as the number of teaching hospitals in each market and the number of ENT specialists. However, as such data were not available for all markets, an analysis of the major population centres of each region would need to be used as a broad approximation of the number of feasible implanting locations.

Possible constraints included the degree to which the size of the required medical and social welfare support team would limit the number of potential implanting sites such teams did not currently exist and their establishment would involve the commitment of substantial monetary and human resources. Another constraint was the degree to which the educational effort involved in introducing the product would limit the market potential at hospital level, at least in the short term. The number of patients each centre could feasibly handle on an annual basis was another consideration.

The third level that would affect market size was the governmental or national level. The promulgation of this type of medical innovation, which involved a high degree of capital expenditure and/or human resource commitment, was critically dependent upon the support of governmental and large private health organisations in any individual market. Expenditure on the health and social services sectors differed between countries and national markets could also be expected to differ in attitude to the introduction of such a device, depending on the wealth of each country. It was necessary to identify primary markets in terms of current health or social services expenditure levels and trends over time.

The degree to which governments or other health organisations could be expected to support the marketing of such an implant was likely to be critically dependent on the current social cost of deafness, measured in terms of both the direct cost in the form of government expenditure and the indirect cost to society at large. For the device to be promoted, it would be necessary to identify the benefit in terms of reduced total social cost from utilisation of the cochlear implant. A cost–benefit analysis would need to be undertaken in each major market area to assess the social value of the innovation.

Further potential constraints to market size at this level included the degree to which regulatory controls could be a limiting factor in regard to national market acceptance of the product. The stance of the US FDA and similar bodies in Europe required detailed investigation. Such constraints were further complicated by the degree to which international standards could limit production and the degree to which existing patents could impinge upon the development of an internationally marketable device.

Another vital area of investigation was potential overseas competition. A number of major research centres were known to be working on the development of implantable hearing devices. Through discussions with the University of Melbourne (UOM) team and review of the literature, seven major centres were identified. There were four in the USA – House Ear Institute in Los Angeles led by William House, Coleman Memorial Lab at the University of California in San Francisco led by Robin Michelson and Michael Merzenich, the Department of Otolaryngology at Stanford Medical Centre in California led by Blair Simmons and co-leader Bob White, and the University of Utah in Salt Lake City led by William Dobelle and Donald Eddington. In Europe, research was being conducted by Service ORL du Centre, Hospitalo-Universitaire, Paris, led by Claude-Henri Chouard and Patrick

MacLeod and by the Department of Otolaryngology at the University of Vienna led by Kurt Burian with Erwin and Ingeborg Hochmair as co-leaders. In the UK the two main groups were University College London led by Adrian Fourcin and Ellis Douek, and at UCH led by Graham Fraser.

Determining the size and progress of the potential competition was information critical to the Nucleus Group decision on whether to pursue the project or leave it to others. If another research group potentially had a better product, then Nucleus would not be interested in wasting its scarce and valuable research and engineering resources.

Yetton and Hirshorn did a thorough literature review of the publications produced by each research group and organised trips to meet each team individually. The literature reviews provided a good background understanding and working knowledge of the pros and cons of each group's research. However, published research usually lags behind the current status of research work by a considerable amount, so the trips would update and supplement published research reviews via personal investigation in each major research centre. The outcome of this market research was expected to be a report focusing on the relative status of competitor groups to the UOM device, which would inform both the Australian government and Nucleus Group decision-making. In particular, the analysis would be focused on the degree to which competitive research would be likely to lead to a commercially marketable product.

Assessment of the competitor groups included a review of each major team in terms of patient numbers and the types and method of selection, funding, surgery, rehabilitation methods and time required, research team size and composition, system design features such as electrodes, receiver and speech processor, current status and future prospects for the research program. The degree to which government or commercial financial support was assisting each development was also a consideration, as was each team's projected time-frame to commercial availability, if that was indeed the goal.

In practice, the potential friction between the two team members was never a huge problem. A good professional, Yetton knew there were 'horses for courses' and she let Hirshorn take the lead when it was appropriate. It was a matter of being pragmatic. She understood that medical researchers might well prefer to be interviewed by another medic, particularly about patient issues. Yetton was free to observe and use her skills as a psychologist and commercial analyst to focus on the team environment and intangibles. She and Hirshorn proved to be a perfect skill match for evaluating the research teams, Hirshorn from a medical and scientific point of view and Yetton playing to her strengths by observing the commercial and personal dynamics. Yetton could assess which of the research teams was really able to come up with the goods, commercially. Were they actually going to be able to find a commercial partner? Were they even interested? Or was their interest more on the research side? Would they actually be able to work with or for a commercial partner? She could spend more time observing and assessing the interpersonal dynamics of the academic teams, determining whether the interviewees had the right skills and formed a well-rounded team. This was no piece of cake, as the teams being interviewed were typically intelligent, ambitious and competitive academics. They weren't going to give much away beyond what was already in the public domain through their research publications. In the main, interviewees were quite cagey. They knew that Yetton and Hirshorn represented the Australian government and were assessing the worldwide potential of the cochlear implant, and they were certainly cognisant of their own commercial prospects. Some researchers were welcoming, in the hope that their device might be recommended instead of the UOM implant.

Yetton and Hirshorn's first destination was the USA. It was a big market and patient funding for the device, through insurance and other means, was available. Several research groups were working on implantable prostheses and there were many excellent hospitals with skilled surgeons. Their initial visit was to Owen Black at the Pittsburgh Eye and Ear Infirmary, followed by a visit to the House Ear Institute. House had always been very open about his work, regularly inviting doctors to come and witness his implant procedure for training purposes. He invited the Nucleus team to come and see him operate and he was certainly the easiest to interview. Confident that he had the best product, he was very relaxed and in the spirit of collaboration invited Hirshorn and Yetton to be in the operating theatre during the next single-channel cochlear implant in a patient. Yetton was nervous. She was not worried about the blood, the skin being peeled back from the face or the noise of the drill burrowing into the skull, but she was very anxious about breaching operating protocols in the theatre. Hirshorn was very helpful. 'Just put your hands behind your back', he said 'and don't move.' Yetton took his advice. No protocols were broken and the operation was quick and impressive.

That was the only operation observed by the team. Unlike the other research teams, House was well established in the USA, had a large and well-funded private clinic (the House Ear Institute) dedicated to his surgery and research and did not consider anyone else to be a real competitor. His single-channel cochlear implant had been very successful and it dominated the embryonic US market. The Australian multi-channel device was in its infancy and House did not consider it any kind of threat.

House's view was understandable. He had trained most of the surgeons in the USA who were interested in cochlear implants and he had a loyal following. Although Graeme Clark was a very careful surgeon, he was extremely slow. Surgery in Clark's theatre took about eight hours whereas House and other surgeons could do it in three to four hours. House was quick, although that was partly because the technology in his implant was simpler. Hirshorn and Yetton didn't think that the House implant was very effective, compared to the Melbourne device. House made no pretence that his device would allow a deaf person to hear speech. It simply improved a deaf person's hearing so that they could hear some sounds, compared to the silence that they had previously lived in. To House and other research groups, that was sufficient improvement. They considered the idea that a deaf person might be able to hear speech and, if pre-lingual, actually learn to speak was no more than wishful thinking.

It took two months to visit all the competitor groups across the USA and Europe. It was not always easy for Yetton at a personal level. She tried to stay in touch with her family via telex and short, very expensive, long-distance phone calls but it was difficult due to the time difference. The interviews were also emotionally draining. The Nucleus team knew it had only one chance to get a full understanding of each research team's achievements and capabilities. They succeeded in interviewing all the research teams and emphasised the comparative evaluation of each team, and included an up-to-date description of each team's research developments and interests.

The last interview was with Clark. This was going to be interesting. Yetton and Hirshorn had made a conscious decision to see him last so that his work could be assessed in the light of the rest of the world's efforts. The trip to Melbourne earlier in the project had just been to get a preliminary overview of the challenge that lay ahead. They hadn't talked with Clark in depth.

Yetton and Hirshorn went through the same interview process with Clark as they had with everyone else, in terms of the results he was getting and meeting his patients. Clark seemed nervous, sitting on the edge of his seat and saying, 'Oh, now we are in for the third degree aren't we?' By this time Yetton and Hirshorn were quite knowledgeable in the field and had probably seen more of the inside workings of the overseas competition than Clark had. Some overseas researchers had been cagey at conferences and it was doubtful that Clark would have been allowed into their laboratories. Yetton and Hirshorn had visual comparisons and were in a good position to judge the UOM cochlear implant.

Nothing they had seen was nearly as sophisticated as Clark's device. Yetton was ready to be convinced because she had seen so many poorer options, and it was abundantly clear that Clark's approach achieved better results for patients. This was key. Yetton considered that Clark's approach was more pragmatic and patient-focused than that of other researchers. For instance, the Hochmairs in Austria clearly had the best electrode – they eventually became a third major force in the industry. Their electrode was certainly better than the one in Melbourne, but there appeared to be disagreement and uncertainty among researchers as to whether more or fewer electrodes would provide the best result. Clark appeared to provide a better answer. He and his team of bio-engineers had experimented with electrodes, putting them in different places and tuning them for the best effect. It seemed that this approach worked better than other frameworks.

The UOM team had demonstrated that more electrodes were better than fewer when comparing the hearing results from the various research teams. Correctly placing the electrodes enabled the audiologists to fine-tune the device so that the patient received a sound combination that allowed them to hear speech. Although all teams used an element of unique patient fine-tuning, some found it very difficult to get it right. Although the market research study had been difficult, Yetton and

Hirshorn could draw a conclusion. The device created by the UOM team, led by Clark, was the best available in the world.

The market size estimates were equally important in determining the overall feasibility assessment and there were literally hundreds of assumptions involved in the production of such estimates. Fortunately, Yetton was highly numerate. She had a quantitative focus and training, but she couldn't do it all. She employed skilled specialists to assist with the number-crunching and putting the story together, including an econometrician from Macquarie University. There was also assistance with sections on patents and regulatory approvals; Yetton had laid a good foundation by developing and defining the final structure of the report. The logic of the report structure was clear but only one person could ultimately put it all together and the task was going to be long and laborious.

Despite the difficulties, the final report was a coherent, logical and sellable story with a concluding section that was vital in determining the commercial direction for the cochlear implant. Should the government invest in this Australian invention? Should the Nucleus Group continue along the path of commercialisation or was the UOM device an interesting experiment that would have little to offer the corporate world?

The study concluded that there was a significant world market for the product, particularly in the USA and Europe. It estimated that about 10% of the profoundly deaf, or about 50 000 patients worldwide, were possible implant candidates. In addition, the data suggested that another 3000 new cases might occur each year worldwide. Although the total number of potential customers may have appeared small, the average price of $10 000 per patient as estimated by the cost plan meant that the total value of the market was substantial. The market study justified the further development of the implant. The report concluded that although there was no clear vision of the ultimate capabilities of multi-channel cochlear implants, it was very clear what a commercially exploitable device must aim to be. It had to be a portable, multi-channel, take-home device backed by a sound rehabilitation program. Its capabilities had to be demonstrably better than those of the existing external vibrotactile devices that were worn on the body (generally on the fingers), powerful high-gain hearing aids and single-channel implants. The prospects for the

UOM device were promising, provided that the necessary and extensive programs of pre-market testing, training and marketing were carried out and an appropriately skilled commercial partner was available.

Putting together credible projections was tricky. It was vital to be absolutely pragmatic about the way the global market dynamics would evolve. In some instances it was necessary to modify the raw projections using judgment rather than science. The estimates needed to consider how many implants could be done, starting with year 1 and showing the growth for each subsequent year. Yetton and Hirshorn had good comparisons from Telectronics' pacemaker sales development which were an enormous help in framing sensible growth projections. The projected trend data indicated that sales would start small and grow slowly. It was expected to start with 10 implants then grind up to 100, taking two to three years to get to significant numbers.

The projections were spot-on. Ten years later Yetton was asked to do a recap on the numbers she had provided. She was completely astonished and somewhat proud to see that the company, and indeed the new industry as a whole, was still using her original projected numbers, which had stood the test of time. That was thrilling. But back in December 1979 she simply delivered the report and left the decision-making process to those higher up the company hierarchy. Having carried out the task that was demanded of her, Yetton went back to her long-postponed day job.

CHAPTER 6.

A prototype became commercially possible: the tiger team

'Watch this, Lois,' instructed Peter Seligman as he waved a coil of wire above another coil to demonstrate to the audiologist a much simplified method of getting power and data across the skin in a secure and efficient way. Two circuit boards the size of paperback books lay on the bench in front of them. A light came on in one of them. 'What is it?' she asked. 'A cochlear implant,' Seligman announced. 'See when I bring this coil close to that one, the light comes on. That light represents an electrode. If I change this switch on the other board, a different light comes on.' 'And', he proudly went on, 'all the power comes from this board, the one that's outside the body.' 'That is a cochlear implant?' the audiologist asked sceptically. 'Well, it's a beginning,' Seligman replied.

It was 1980 and patents for a commercial cochlear implant device had been registered, a costing plan had been developed and a market study identifying a substantial market for the Melbourne device had been completed. Telectronics really needed to make a decision whether to tender for the project or walk away from it. Paul Trainor, CEO of the Nucleus Group, was very keen and David Money had also become convinced that it was a challenge worth pursuing. Jim Loughman, then CEO of Telectronics, was doubtful about the long term, realising that it would turn Telectronics in a very different direction. The French company Synthelab, a major shareholder of Telectronics, made it clear that the cochlear implant did not have enough in common with the cardiac treatment in which it was interested, so that meant that Telectronics would not be able to tender for the government grant to commercialise the cochlear device. Nucleus was not appropriate because it wasn't an operating company, it was just a holding company for the Nucleus Group, but it was the best alternative until a new cochlear division could be established. Thus, Nucleus took on the role of the bidding company.

Therefore it was Nucleus and not Telectronics that undertook the negotiations with the government for Phase 2 of the project and ultimately arrived at a successful bid. There really wasn't much choice. Although a number of firms bid for the tender, Nucleus, given its experience with medical devices, was the only real option in Australia to undertake such a project. Phase 2 of the project required Nucleus to engineer the bionic ear and to make it smaller and more reliable. The University of Melbourne (UOM) team committed to further develop speech-processing strategies, as well as surgical and training programs for the US clinics and biological safety studies.

On 28 October 1981, Trainor announced that Money, who he described as the first applicant for the position, had been chosen to lead the project. Trainor also announced that the selection of Money's lieutenants was vital, particularly for the early phase of the project. Nucleus had chosen two competent and complementary people to assist Money in leading the project – Jim Patrick from the UOM and Peter Crosby, who had spent the last three years as director of Northern Metropolitan Regional Biomedical Engineering Services. Money would begin with the new subsidiary on a part-time basis from Telectronics; he was the first member of what became known as Trainor's 'tiger team'. Chris Daly, who had worked with Money to develop the new commercial design, stayed with Telectronics and did not join the Cochlear team. In Sydney the Cochlear team also involved David Cowdery and Carl Doring as consultants. Via Nucleus, the team co-opted Mike Hirshorn on FDA, patents and preliminary clinical trials. The administrative and financial support was provided by Robert Foot, Aileen Wilson, Touchique Siepa and Liz Noonan.

Money was cautious of too much enthusiasm and from the beginning was determined that Nucleus needed an ongoing commitment from the UOM, to ensure that any negotiations for licence fees would not provide a basis of future legal action. Also critical for success was the availability of know-how and ongoing UOM research, for which Nucleus was paying a licence fee. Money let it be known that a transfer of personnel would be essential for a quick commercial outcome. Trainor, cognisant of the impact that staff losses would have on Graeme Clark who was still very much a part of the second phase of the program, asked Clark's permission to approach the UOM team. For Clark, this was a difficult decision. Losing key people was a blow to the UOM team's ability to meet its obligations for the grant and to do further research. However, losing the possibility to progress the research to successful commercialisation could derail the whole process, so he agreed. He was grateful to have been asked, and at least he now had additional financial resources with which to hire new staff. He also still had a strong skill base with Joe Tong (speech engineering and psychophysics), Ray Black (neurophysiology) and Peter Blamey (psychophysics). Also on the team in Melbourne were Peter Seligman (signal processing), Grant da Costa (signal processing), Lois Martin (audiology), Richard Dowell (audiology), Rob Shepherd (animal studies) and Christine Bunn (administration). The Melbourne group also had the services of two surgeons, Brian Pyman and Robert Webb, who worked on a sessional basis.

With Clark's blessing, the Sydney team approached Patrick to become the first of Money's lieutenants. Patrick had been project manager during the development of the prototype and had all the right attributes to manage the knowledge and prejudices of the UOM team. Before accepting his position with Clark, Patrick had asked what it would lead to in the future. Clark could not give him a definite answer but replied that it could lead to the implant being developed commercially and that Patrick would be able to work in industry. That was Patrick's preferred option. He had no ambitions to remain in academia, therefore he happily accepted the offer of moving to Sydney. His move to the commercial group, however, left a vacuum in the Melbourne team. According to the licensing agreement, the UOM had a lot of deliverables to get Nucleus up and running. Rob Shepherd was approached to move into the role and did a magnificent job of managing the team after Patrick's departure. With skill and enthusiasm, he was able to manage and coordinate the engineering, clinical and software efforts of the team. Each time a new implant, electrode or speech-coding strategy was introduced, Shepherd carried out the crucial safety studies without which it would be impossible to achieve FDA approval.

In Sydney, the recruiting for commercial development began in earnest. Nucleus advertised Australia-wide a number of positions that would provide essential project skills. Among others, it managed to attract Leo Port, who had come to Australia from Russia in 1975 without much English. The USSR had been pressured by the USA to allow people of various ethnic origins to leave the USSR if that was their wish. Port's parents were from one of the targeted ethnic regions, so he took the opportunity to leave the communist régime although it meant abandoning his engineering studies at university.

Immigrating to Australia with only $US90 – all he was allowed to take out of the USSR – he found work quickly. He was forever grateful for his first job in Australia. Only two weeks after arriving Port started work for a lift company as an electrician, without speaking English. His interview panel had included a Hungarian supervisor who knew a few Russian words. In the interview the Hungarian had pointed to a circuit board on which Port identified a transformer, a word which was the same in Russian and English. With a few more words he impressed the employer and got the job. That was very lucky, but he was even luckier to be put to work with a sympathetic young Australian who spoke only English. They communicated using sign language.

After a year, in 1976, Port felt that he had enough language skills and started studying electrical engineering at a technical college. At the end of the semester he achieved 100% in every subject – he decided it was too easy, so he dropped out and waited until the beginning of the next academic year to start a degree in electrical engineering. It was not easy. He took notes in Russian, then had to come home and try to translate them into English. It was incredibly inefficient and took an extraordinary amount of time. Eventually he learnt to do it all in English although his spelling was never very good. As time went on he picked up more language and in 1977 university fees were abolished. This made life a lot easier.

The improvement in his financial and language positions allowed him to get a job teaching electrical engineering at a college level. It was a very heavy load: he was going to university at night, teaching three days a week and for the other two days was working towards a diploma of education. He achieved the diploma with bare passes, a reflection of the time he could devote to it. It took only three years before Port began to look to the future. He was becoming a little bored with teaching the same topics repetitively although he was still progressing well with his degree. By that time he was married and had one daughter. His wife noticed an advertisement in the national newspaper, the *Australian*; it was unusual because job advertisements in Sydney were usually in the *Sydney Morning Herald*. Port thought the ad was pretty bizarre. It showed a Leonardo da Vinci drawing of a human male stretched out and it said barely anything about the job. It did, however, say that the company was looking for scientists, engineers and technicians to work on some advanced engineering and it sounded interesting.

Port went for an interview. A panel of Money, Patrick, Loughman and a couple of others all sat at a long table facing Port, who was alone on the other side. This did not intimidate him because he wasn't desperate for a job; he still had his teaching job at TAFE. His initial intention was to attend the interview for practice and to see what kind of job was being offered. While they chatted the door opened and a very confident man walked in. Port quickly realised that it was Trainor. It was obvious that he was an important person in the room, made particularly evident by the reaction of the others. He said, 'Five of you and this poor guy sitting on this side of the table. I am going to sit next to him.' Trainor accompanied Port on his side of the table and said, 'Now ask your questions.' They all laughed and eventually Trainor left the room.

Trainor was very good at assessing people quickly and didn't need to stay for the technical discussion. The panel asked nothing about Port's experience or technological knowledge. He asked exactly what the company would be doing. The advertisement had been a Nucleus ad and they replied, 'Well, we have a number of companies and we are looking broadly how we can bring people with good energy into the company. One of the companies that we will be starting is the bionic ear.' At this time a program called the 'Six Million Dollar Man', about a man with replacement bionic body parts, was on television and Port thought, 'Are these people for real?' They talked about the topic only briefly; when Port came home he told his wife, 'They are a strange lot and they are talking about the "Six Million Dollar Man" stuff with hearing. I don't think it was serious.' Two or three weeks later he received a call to come for another interview, this time with only Money and Patrick. That interview was very technical and focused on the cochlear implant. There were written questions and discussion of some technical problems, which Port could handle well because he was still in his final year of university and thus was reasonably up-to-date.

However, he left the interview not knowing how he went. A couple of weeks later he was offered the job. The company would pay less than he was already earning but he decided to accept the job because it appeared to offer better opportunities in the longer term although he still had no real idea of what he would actually be doing.

Little did Port know that he was exactly the kind of person the advertisement had hoped to attract: someone who had the intelligence and drive to go from not speaking a language to teaching engineering at a TAFE level while completing a university engineering degree in a foreign language – all in the space of three years. That took very focused hard work as well as intelligence. The company was seeking someone who would be interested in thinking outside the square, who would be excited rather than afraid of challenges that appeared to be impossible.

Nucleus also advertised for a mechanical or materials engineer who would be responsible for the construction of the implant package. It appointed Janusz Kuzma, who had recently arrived in Australia, as another member of the team. Kuzma had come to Australia from Poland in 1981 just before Lech Walesa's trade union uprising. It was good timing and Kuzma had expected to continue his career in high technology. He quickly discovered that in Australia, high-tech did not exist. Most of the innovative technologies were stripped and shipped overseas and most of the Australian electronic companies, as far as he could see, were involved with reselling things that had been made in Taiwan or China. Kuzma found work quickly but in companies that were not what he considered to be high-tech, and he was far from happy. Then he came across the Nucleus advertisement in the newspaper and responded, without any idea what it was referring to. He had no experience in the medical field nor did he know anything about the biotechnical field, but he was an expert in the field of hermetically sealed packages for the semiconductor industry. During the interview, Patrick asked what Kuzma considered to be some tricky questions on how he would solve various problems. Kuzma gave the answers that he knew Patrick wanted to hear, and hoped for the best.

He got the job but it took him a few weeks to work out what a cochlea was. There was no equivalent in the Polish dictionary and he was afraid to ask anyone in case he lost the job. He didn't want to lose the opportunity to work on this interesting project that was supposed to stimulate a cochlea. After a few weeks he had worked out what the project involved and what he had to do, in a general way. He was lucky that some of his knowledge was new to Australia, so he looked knowledgeable. The project gave Kuzma the opportunity to learn a new profession in biomedical engineering. Although initially he didn't know what they meant by reliability, biocompatibility and precious metals, the challenge was exciting and a lot of luck was on his side when everything worked the first time around.

Peter Seligman did not join the tiger team. Like Patrick, he had been part of the University of Melbourne team and he continued to work for the UOM until January 1983. However, unlike Patrick, he had convinced the company that he should work from Melbourne. Given Money's determination to have good connections with Melbourne no one had a problem with that proposal and in 1980 Seligman demonstrated to audiologist Lois Martin the idea that the whole of the receiver (at least the implanted part) could be implemented on a single low-power chip.

The expression 'tiger team' was Trainor's. He defined it as a small A-grade team with one goal and full-time commercial commitment. As was his way, he created competitive tension and gave the team an absolutely free hand. In essence, there appeared to be two tiger teams. The core group consisted of the first three people employed for the project with a Trainor dollar incentive to produce the prototype on his schedule, then there was the rest of the group. The tension later exploded in a number of ways, but for the first few years while the company was in its infancy it was a fantastic experience for everyone involved. They had focus and enthusiasm and there was testosterone everywhere. They worked hard and enjoyed it, not stepping on each other's toes or trying to push each other around as can happen in a larger company. It was definitely a good team. Trainor stayed in the background, watching and supervising, but people felt that they had control. There was freedom to use new approaches and not be bound by the conventions of a larger, older group. There was also freedom to investigate tangents that sometimes really paid off. The outcome was that a small group of people worked together and developed components of systems that were unique. Systems that had never been done before or so well. Everything in the puzzle fitted together.

Port experienced the freedom early. His first day at the company was in September 1981, which was also the last day that a permanent facility space was available in

Telectronics for the new division. After the decision to form the cochlear group, Telectronics cleared one of the rooms in its R&D facility. Port introduced himself; the staff pointed to the end of the corridor and said, 'Last door on the right.' He entered a room that was approximately 3×4 m and almost completely empty. There was nothing there except for two telephone books on the floor and a telephone sitting on top of them. Port's confidence faltered and he thought, 'My God, what have I done?' However, within minutes Money came into the room and made him feel very welcome. A few minutes later Patrick also walked in and the three men had the first unofficial meeting of the new company.

A-graders don't get intimidated easily. Port began to order desks, microscopes and anything else necessary for the research. He formed useful relationships with different suppliers and made a big effort to get to know Telectronics staff who understood manufacturing – there was no one else who had the experience to do the kind of purchasing that he needed to ask about. He became the Head of Manufacturing and built the department from absolute scratch, starting in that empty room.

On the heels of the newcomers, Trevor Marshall joined the company. Marshall was instrumental in developing the electronic design for the diagnostic and programming unit and was involved with the digital/logical part of the interface with the computer. He was a very strong digital designer. He didn't stay for very long, moving to exciting grounds in Silicon Valley, but he was a major influence on Port and gave him a lasting interest in computers. Port was specialising in electronic instrumentation in his electrical engineering degree. They used computers at the university but not at this level. Marshall brought boxes of computer magazines from home to encourage Port's knowledge and lasting interest in computers at a time well before IBM personal computers. The Cochlear Division had no computer development, computer repair or computer management department for about 15 years; it had just one person, Port. Because he showed interest in it Marshall mentored him like a young protégé, providing a lot of practical experience that Port would never have been able to get from his university lecturers, who were well behind Marshall's level of knowledge. Port also worked closely with Patrick and Crosby and sometimes with Seligman, focusing on developing, building and trying out equipment to be used for testing and improving the implantable and external components of the system.

Patrick was very much involved with the big picture. Crosby focused mostly on the speech processor interface and the software which allowed the programming computer to communicate with the patient's speech processor. The first version of the software had been written by Jonathon Ridler at the UOM. It was written in Basic, an interpreter language, but the project used a more elaborate version that could be compiled into executable code that could run by itself. Crosby managed to contract Andrew Mortlock from the Australian National University to work on Ridler's version of the software. Mortlock worked on the program full-time for about nine months, then part-time for about 15 months. To his delight, Patrick offered him a full-time job on staff at the end of 1985. When the company began to use IBM personal computers, Mortlock rewrote the programming software from Basic to a more professional language, C, which could use the ever-increasing memory in each new generation of computers. It took about nine months before the software could be used in the clinic.

While Port was developing his computer skills, Kuzma, the mechanical engineer, was designing the miniaturised implantable package. Essentially the implant consisted of four components – the hermetic package that housed the electronics, a coil to pick up data and power from the external transmitter, the electrode array and a group of feed-throughs to bring the electrical connections from inside the package to the electrode wires outside.

The initial idea was that the hermetic package would be ceramic, to allow the radio-frequency magnetic field from the transmitter to couple to the receiver coil. Kuzma promoted the idea of a titanium device like that used in the Telectronics pacemaker, although the pacemaker was much bigger. He carefully studied the Telectronics device, with its sophisticated use of titanium and its hermetic sealing technology, then significantly developed and enhanced that system for use in the cochlear device. The enclosure was reasonably easy to make from metal and easy to weld together, but there was the question of how to get an electrical signal in and out of the device.

This was a big issue. Pacemakers have only a few outputs, two to perhaps four. Kuzma was told that the cochlear implant would need maybe 10, maybe 15, maybe more outputs. He suggested what some thought was absolutely crazy – the idea of putting platinum tubes into green ceramic before firing them. But it worked, and was the solution for the fourth of the four components.

However, the metal case was a problem because the cochlear implant needed to receive power and data from the outside world. The coil had to be outside the package so that it would not be shielded by the metal. A number of turns of fine wire were required. This was a weak point since there was potential for breakage of the wire, short circuits between turns, and leakage of current in the hostile biological environment. One idea to overcome this problem involved putting the wires in a platinum tube, but that would have shunted away the magnetic field. However, since the platinum tube was a single-turn coil, the wires in the tube were not required. The use of a voltage transformer was a solution to the problem.

The big advantage of using a transformer was that the external coil could be constructed with just one turn. This made it very robust, since the wire was braided. The low voltage meant that any electrical leakage was minimised. In bench tests, the pair of coil connections (feed-throughs) could be put in a puddle of saline with almost no change in receiver voltage. A single turn also meant that there was no possibility of a short circuit between two turns. In spite of the concerns about the power loss of such a tiny transformer, it turned out to be an efficient enough solution to the second component. In fact, it was so practical that the system was still in use in 2012.

The third component – the electrode array – was, according to the company, an issue that had already been decided as per the UOM model. Kuzma considered this to be absolutely wrong. Although the structure of the electrode was decided, the method of fabrication was unwieldy to say the least. It took a gifted jeweller, Geoff Lavery, about a week to build a single electrode array. Kuzma built the electrode in his own way and cooked it in the oven at home. It smelt like chicken but it worked really well. Kuzma was not one of the core tiger team. He knew that they were on a better financial deal and believed that he was incredibly underpaid, so he thought to use his development as leverage to get a better deal. He was convinced that a commercial cochlear implant could not exist without the array that he had designed and delivered.

By now he knew the challenges facing the project and understood that there was no other alternative which they could get in the specified time-frame. It was not just a case of not enough money – there was no one else who could provide it. It was not like writing a purchase order to buy an electrode. This was different. The device eventually had 22 outputs but the electrode had become much more complex. Every contact more than proportionately escalated the complexity of the process. It was a new product on the market and was 10 times more complex than anything else that was currently available. The technology was excellent and a huge improvement on all that had been done before in implantable electronics.

Kuzma had made the prototypes himself, so he knew what was required and what it would do. He had given parts of the development to people who worked closely with him, and heard them complaining that it was impossible, too difficult, crazy. But Kuzma had a very good and versatile team from technicians to toolmakers, a small orchestra that put together the whole. Before Kuzma approached Money, he knew exactly what he was dealing with.

Kuzma reported to Money and presented his new package design but, instead of receiving accolades, Money looked at him and showed no interest. Kuzma had not been asked to do this. His job was to build ceramic feed-throughs. Money was a little shocked at the behaviour of this newcomer, barging into his office and demanding recognition for something out of left field. But Kuzma was determined and, since he was not getting anywhere with the negotiation, he grabbed the package from the table and walked out the door. As he went out he shouted, 'You guys can pack your bags and go home because this project is dead!'

Money was very professional, very smart, extremely honest, well-respected and well-liked. He avoided conflict, always tried to resolve issues in a methodical way and therefore provided stability to the whole project. His professionalism was instrumental in preventing or minimising explosions. On this occasion Money reacted differently from how most people would – he just got over the superficial insults and it never became an issue that Kuzma was not highly polished in his behaviour. Others may not have reacted so objectively, which could have led to a less favourable ending for Kuzma or the company. Money gave the Polish engineer a chance to settle down then called him at home, asking him to come back. Kuzma came back the same afternoon. Kuzma was instrumental in finding a revolutionary but practical way to reliably build 22 electrodes and bring their connections out of a titanium electronics package through a ceramic seal.

Throughout late 1981 and 1982 there were 18 months of feverish activity in which the entire system was redesigned from the ground up. The pace and progress were breathtaking. A new single-chip implant was designed and packaged in a titanium case. The speech processor was further miniaturised by using hybrid technology (a mixture of chips and conventional components) for the analog circuits and a single chip for the digital part. Tasks that would normally take a year were done in weeks. In 18 months two silicon chips and two hybrid circuits were developed, packaged in boxes, tested and fitted to six patients and the testing was completed on the patients.

Seligman was instrumental in designing the circuitry of the speech processor, the externally worn part of the cochlear implant system. Patrick, who was by then working in Sydney, returned to Melbourne on a regular basis for a few days at a time. Their ideas were mostly tossed around during telephone conversations. In Sydney Money worked with Daly on the clever analog circuitry in the implant chip, while Patrick created the digital part and radio-frequency link. The burst-duration based control was elegant engineering at its best. It was a masterpiece of simplicity and robustness.

As far as stimulation via the electrodes was concerned, simplicity was again the key. Charge balance, essential for the safety of the cochlea, was achieved by using a single current source and flipping the electrode connections. This, together with the idea of shorting (connecting) all the electrodes together after each stimulation pulse, gave maximum safety without the use of bulky coupling capacitors.

When Patrick came to Melbourne they discussed circuit ideas and Seligman would start wire-wrapping a prototype almost immediately, to be bench-tested within a few days. Although much work still needed to be done, a large part of the design was born then. The decisions made in those weeks resulted in a device which remained the current clinical product until 1997. The potential of the device still provides improved performance. Patrick and Seligman complemented each other perfectly and often thought that it would indeed be rare to see a more productive working relationship.

Port was in charge of manufacturing the speech processors, the externally worn part of the cochlear implant system. The processor consisted of two analog hybrid circuits used for analysing sound and a digital encoder for transmitting the information to the implant. A radio-frequency driver supplied power and data to the patient-worn coil. The manufacturing details of the speech processor, the computer interface and the ultraviolet light source to erase and reprogram the patient's speech processor were put together by Crosby.

Seligman developed a system called the EMU (electrode monitor unit), which was a functional test of the external system. A second version was called the ostrich (as a joke – an emu is a large Australian bird). This device took information from the speech processor after it had been processed by the front end, and resynthesised the digital output into the sounds representing the sound that a patient might hear.

The signal input for the speech processor hybrid circuit manufacturer's test system was a device used as a speech therapy trainer. Essentially it was a tape recorder without the tape. Instead of the tape, a magnetic stripe on a paper card was used. The team in Melbourne would record sentences such as, 'The little grey blankets lay around on the floor.' Port still remembered the test sentences, 27 years later. The sentences were composed to contain different sets of syllables and different consonants and vowels. Although the result was a very confused static sound, it was possible to understand whether the electronics worked. It was also possible to start fault-finding. Basically, it was possible to hear a crude rendition of what the deaf person was hearing. After listening to the test sentence cards for a few weeks, Port thought that it no longer sounded like a crude rendition. In fact, it was becoming so natural that it was possible to hear the differences between the various processors. Seligman and Port would confirm patients' claims about processors not sounding right. The fact that after a while they could understand the recordings without effort and could differentiate the quality of the sound was another proof that patients could adapt to what was to them a 'new' sound, all due to the amazing plasticity of the brain.

As a final production functionality test of the overall speech processor, an early Texas Instruments toy, the Speak and Spell, was used as a speech synthesiser to provide the test signal. The Speak and Spell was set to make a certain utterance, which was fed through the speech processor. The stimulated electrodes were output via the EMU to a computer and the electrode stimulation pattern was compared with a template in the computer. If the pattern of stimulation fell within the template boundaries, the speech processor had passed the test.

The first Nucleus cochlear implant used a wire headband to hold the external coil in place over the implanted coil. The use of a pair of magnets was discussed but there was too little time for safety tests which could confirm whether the blood vessels in the tissue between the magnets would be too constricted. Kuzma was instrumental in designing the headset which was made in-house by Port's team. It was a very important part of the overall system and was a lightweight headphone-like arrangement that sat over the top or around the back of the head. Alignment between the external and implanted coils was essential – as soon as the headpiece was 1 cm off-centre, the link and thus the implant stopped working. An additional difficulty was that the headset was constantly shifted by head movements, its wires bending in every direction. To fit a headset, the clinician had to carefully bend the wires so that the coil sat in the right place. It never did. It always needed a bit more bending. When it was just right, inevitably the wires would break and the headset, including the microphone, would be unusable.

Ken Dormer, a clinician in Oklahoma who had been fitting the House single-channel device, was also struggling with coil alignment. Drawing from the dental field, he suggested using a pair of magnets, one in the centre of the implanted coil and the other in the centre of the external coil, to hold the external coil in place. He patented the idea and gave the patent to the Baptist Medical Centre of Oklahoma. The Oklahoma patent became an obstacle when the tiger team came to implement the idea of the magnet. They approached the assignee and asked if they could use the licence. They were offered the use of the intellectual property at a cost of $1000 per magnet. This was outrageous; on consultation, the Nucleus patent lawyers advised that they could use it after all. They did so, with excellent results.

The diagnostic/programming unit consisted of the speech processor interface, the computer and special software. It was the interface between the audiologist and the speech processor. It was also, however, a victim of hasty design. Clinicians were plagued by problems when erasing patient 'maps' from the speech processor when they needed to be changed. The process was a major operational problem. There was an agonising wait (with a deaf person) while the old map was being erased. It was supposed to take only a few minutes but instead took half an hour. The circuitry to drive the UV lamp was seriously underpowered, and attempts to increase it had the side effect of drawing so much current from the supply rail that the interface frequently crashed. It would be easy today to criticise the apparently sloppy design and the lack of testing and verification that prevailed in those days, but it was the drive to do whatever it took to get to the objective that worked. On the external side of the system it was a 'no holds barred' approach. On the implanted side, safety and reliability were always viewed as vital.

So determined was the group to succeed that whenever there was a potential problem, they went to multiple vendors. The project could not go ahead if either of the two silicon chip developments were delayed or failed. Chip development was critical, so they went to two companies for both the implant chip and the speech processor data encoder. They used the product from the first company to successfully produce the goods; the other company was very slow and the project could have been very much delayed if the group had relied on only that vendor.

The team talked to three vendors concerning the analog hybrid circuits, but placed an order with only one. The first possibility was a Sydney-based company, represented by two chain-smokers with whom the team couldn't envisage working. Their very makeshift approach was uninspiring. The tiger team preferred a Melbourne company which seemed much more professional and which had an advanced, multi-layer approach. However, it had continual supply and reliability problems. A third would-be vendor made some unsuccessful prototypes (the device didn't fit in the box), so the tiger team returned to the first vendor. The chain-smokers won after all.

The configuration of the new Nucleus device was such that the stimulation could occur on any of 22 electrodes with the remaining electrodes acting as a return path. Compared to the UOM system, this doubled the number of channels without needing more bands on the electrode array. Furthermore, a bipolar mode allowed current to be passed between any two electrode bands, without the use of a common ground.

The idea of using purely intra-cochlear (bipolar) stimulation came from the physiologists, whose animal experiments had found that monopolar stimulation caused so much current spread that the facial nerve was stimulated as well as the auditory nerve. Hence, monopolar stimulation was considered unsuitable. A decade or so later, however, it was realised that although this was a problem with the stimulation in lab cats it did not apply to humans. The eventual conversion to monopolar stimulation resulted in a reduction, by a factor of 6, in the amount of electrical charge needed to stimulate. The additional current spread did not cause any reduction in patient results.

By the time the team was designing the commercial device, they knew that simultaneous stimulation of a number of electrodes was not required and in fact was rather a liability. The new stimulator had only one current source, which was simply switched to the electrode pair to be stimulated. When the opposite charge was applied to maintain current balance, the current source was used again, just switched in with the connections reversed.

The importance of charge balance in electrical stimulation of biological tissues was well recognised and the final safeguard was the shorting of all electrodes together after each pair of stimulation pulses. This was Money's idea, previously used in a pacemaker, to allow stimulating electrodes to be used for recording, shortly after delivering a pulse. Very importantly, it meant that none of the intra-cochlear electrodes needed an isolating capacitor.

The resulting implant stimulator was a masterpiece of elegance and simplicity. The electronics for it were first used in a stimulator called the 'standard' implant, the CS. The device was a single-chip solution, based on a CMOS gate array adapted from a Telectronics array designed by Amalgamated Wireless Australia Micro-electronics, Money's former employer. The implant electronics comprised only this chip with six discrete components. The same electronics were used in the 'Mini' or CI22 implant, as it was later called. No one ever imagined that this device would be implanted in 17 000 recipients.

During the design, development and production of the first systems for the preliminary clinical trials in Melbourne, Money became concerned at the probability of a very long cash drought if the company had to wait years for government approval for each potential market. Cash was always a concern in Nucleus and at this stage the company could not be sure that Australian government support would continue. Money knew that drug companies usually gave free samples for the clinical trials of their new products, but Nucleus could not afford to do so. After the first six trial patients, subsequent patients paid for their cochlear implant.

The time-frame to achieve all the objectives of Phase 2 was extremely short. It was September 1981 by the time the tiger team was in place and by mid 1982 the Nucleus implant had reached the final design stages before implantation. The first Australian implant of the Nucleus design was on 12 September 1982, on Graham Carrick. It was an extraordinary achievement to successfully complete so much so quickly in something that was so complex. Having achieved successful results with the first patient, further implants were undertaken in Melbourne and by the end of 1982 the required six patients had had the newly designed device successfully implanted, with very favourable results. This successful initial trial in Australia gave Nucleus the green light to start the clinical trial in the USA and Europe.

A letter by Trainor, announcing the cochlear project and nominating the people involved, said, 'Thus we aim to attain the impossible by completing Phase 2 in December 1982, that is, to go from the experimental prototype to the completion of preliminary clinical trials.' The objective was achieved. The 'impossible' task was completed one month ahead of schedule.

The brilliance of the development can be expressed in Professor Peter Seligman's words. 'What we experienced in the development of the cochlear implant was something that was beyond our wildest dreams. It was, and still is, a charmed project, in which everything always turned out better than one could have reasonably expected. It wasn't just a once in a lifetime experience; it was a once in many lifetimes experience.'

CHAPTER 7

Proof for the regulators: Mike Hirshorn and Dianne Mecklenburg

Paul Trainor always insisted that if commercialisation of the cochlear implant were to proceed, a separate subsidiary would be established to produce and market the implant. This was consistent with the Nucleus philosophy and structure implied by the company's name. The reasoning behind a separate company structure, Trainor argued, 'was that it gives the independence required for rapid, unencumbered growth but also allows the subsidiary to benefit from the expertise and resources of the parent, Nucleus'. The structure also potentially enabled the attraction of additional shareholders. Nexus Biomedical (soon renamed Cochlear Pty Ltd) was set up as a wholly owned subsidiary company of Nucleus in 1983.

Michael Hirshorn was recruited by Trainor to the Nucleus Group in 1978, initially to Telectronics and then to Cochlear from 1981. Having successfully completed the market study with Maria Yetton in 1979, he stood in the Nucleus boardroom in 1983 struggling with what he had just heard. 'Take this cheque for $10 000 and establish Cochlear Corporation in the US,' Trainor told him. 'Where shall I establish it?' asked Hirshorn. 'Oh, wherever you can be successful' was the short answer. 'But I have a girlfriend,' lamented Hirshorn. 'I am sure you will handle it' was the unsympathetic reply. This was not going to be simple. The Telectronics office was in Denver and that would be Hirshorn's base, but the international networks that had been established over the years for devices such as pacemakers and ultrasound did not extend to ear, nose and throat (ENT) surgeons. This was crucial, because Hirshorn's first task was setting up the subsidiary to gain FDA approval and market the implant in the USA, then Europe and the Middle East.

Nucleus had always expected the company to have three 'legs' to the cochlear implant market and that approximately 40% of demand would be in the USA. Hirshorn was sent there first as the USA was the obvious place to start for a language-related product. At that time the regulatory environment was more advanced in the USA than in other places; Europe looked to the USA for regulatory approval of new products. Hirshorn's medical background gave him the right kind of expertise for the task and, during the world market study in 1979, he and Yetton had established and developed successful relationships with clinics and experts in the ENT field. Many of those who had participated in the study had retained very favourable impressions of Hirshorn, which they reported to the US government. The impressive reports on the survey team formed a good beginning from which to expand.

One of the first people with whom Hirshorn made contact was Dianne Mecklenburg, an audiologist with extensive qualifications. She had experience in cochlear implants and rehabilitation skills for all ages, having worked in the school for the deaf, the Veterans Association and the Otological Medical Group (now the House Ear Institute). She had qualifications in hearing science and speech pathology and as a therapist had been doing work in psychological and speech therapy. All these areas of expertise came together very nicely in the work with cochlear implants.

Mecklenburg had been sponsored to teach at the Lincoln Institute of Health Sciences in Melbourne but was not enjoying her teaching job. It was at an introductory level and not what she wanted so she started sending her résumé to various organisations. Eventually she heard of a group of people doing cochlear implants. Mecklenburg had always believed in cochlear implant technology and, given her experience working with patients for the House/Urban cochlear implant team in the USA, thought that she could teach the Australians something about the technology. She soon realised, however, that she was talking to a team of dynamic people who were far more advanced in multi-channel cochlear implant concepts than any she had seen before. The University of Melbourne (UOM) team offered her a job; she agreed to take a cut in salary and paid back her sponsorship money so that she could begin teaching audiology at the UOM. There she met David Money, who recommended that she work as a consultant for Cochlear when she returned to the

USA. Hirshorn therefore had an excellent contact when he arrived in the USA to set up a new subsidiary for Cochlear.

Hirshorn and Mecklenburg worked together to evaluate potential centres and make contact with key decision-makers in the field. It was also necessary to decide if the centres should be in cities where there would be a larger population of deaf people, or in special centres in smaller cities. In Australia all the centres were in big cities but this was not the case in the USA. Would teams be able to manage people for lengthy rehabilitation sessions if they came from other parts of the USA? Mecklenburg's and Hirshorn's contacts decided the location of some of the centres, and they developed criteria to assess the reputation and proficiency level of surgeons and their multi-skilled teams. Professor Graeme Clark also provided research support and suggested US contacts when required.

The number of contacts required for this exercise was extensive. Sympathetic ENT surgeons were the first group to contact. Although cochlear implant work is now generally considered to be day surgery (the patient goes home the same day), there is always a risk involved. Therefore, surgeons who are well-trained and highly skilled are critical to the success of the implant. In a new industry such as this, it was also necessary to inspire the ENT surgeons to become the medical champions to promote the benefits. The conversion process was not always easy.

But the surgery is not the end of the story. After one to four weeks of healing, the implant is turned on (activated) and programmed for the individual patient. Results are typically not immediate. Post-implantation therapy is required, as well as time for the brain to adapt to hearing new sounds, so audiologists and speech therapists are also critical. In children the therapy can take years, and the participation of the child's family in working on spoken language development can be even more important than therapy. Professionals involved in the implant process thus include speech-language pathologists, auditory-verbal therapists, paediatric audiologists, teachers of the deaf with specialisation in oral deaf education, psychologists and general practitioners. Mecklenburg and Hirshorn needed to identify appropriate professionals in all those areas, inspire them with the new technology, then train and monitor them to obtain rigorous data which could be supplied to the FDA for approval of the implant.

Access to appropriate contacts was made a little easier by networking strategies that had been established earlier. Mecklenburg had some really good contacts in the industry, people she had met while writing her PhD. In the years leading up to the trials, Clark had gathered an impressive list of disciples in the ENT field. As early as 1977, he had strategically invited Jim Jerger, a pioneer in audiology from Baylor Medical College, to be guest of honour at the UOM's inaugural audiology workshop. Baylor Medical College had two outstanding ear surgeons, Bob Alford and Herman Jenkins, whom Clark considered to be ideal future contacts. Such thinking proved absolutely correct – Baylor was one of the first centres in the USA to trial the Nucleus device. Similarly, Brian McCabe, Professor of Otolaryngology at the University of Iowa, had been invited to present a paper at the UOM annual audiology conference in 1981. On hearing Clark speak at the conference, McCabe became very enthusiastic about using the Melbourne device in a comparative study he was planning to undertake. In Iowa, Bruce Gantz was one of the first to undertake US trials of the new device. Once the FDA gave its approval for the trials to begin, Iowa and Baylor Medical College were the first centres in the USA to implant the Nucleus bionic ear. Other surgeons to participate in the US clinical trials were Charlie Mangham from the Mason Clinic in Seattle, Noel Cohen at New York University, George Lyons from the Louisiana State University in New Orleans, Owen Black from the Good Samaritan Hospital in Portland and Julian Nedzelski from the University of Toronto.

Mecklenburg, employed as a consultant, coordinated the various professionals and began to bring the pivotal study together. Hirshorn joined her in April 1984. His main responsibility was to promote the UOM/Nucleus device to a market that did not always recognise or trust Australian scientific excellence. 'There was always the problem of not being American.' Selling the concept of the multi-channel device and its benefits to the US market was difficult due to local competition. Specifically, the 3M/House device was promoted by the very eminent and respected Bill House who spoke at conferences and had trained many of the ENT surgeons. 3M had commenced its trials for FDA approval much earlier, which meant that Cochlear Corporation was lagging behind 3M at this stage. The task of signing up US centres for the trials was made challenging by the fact that, as the 1979 market survey by Telectronics concluded, the UOM group was 'not well known or understood elsewhere' and that an Australian device entering a US market to compete with US devices must start at a disadvantage. It was also frustrating that Clark did not want to travel to the USA, as that constrained the Cochlear team's promotional efforts.

In October 1984, Ginger Minelli, Hirshorn's assistant and Judy Brimacombe, an audiologist and Mecklenburg's assistant, also joined the team. Certain personality characteristics were necessary for the team to succeed in its aims. Colleagues described Hirshorn as very bright and sincere with a very high level of integrity, but very much an opportunistic business entrepreneur driven to succeed. Although working as a consultant, Mecklenburg was very committed to the project. Her major challenge was to develop the protocol that all surgeons, audiologists and clinics would adhere to for a pivotal study that would provide data for FDA approval. Experienced clinicians were recruited rather than salespeople, their experience allowing them to give information and training to potential customers. Specific training courses were instituted for audiologists and otologists (ear surgeons). Emphasis was placed on a team approach to patient care and maximum clinical benefit, and a spirit of selling a philosophy rather than a product was developed. Mecklenburg held training workshops and ran around the USA troubleshooting technical problems. She went to conferences and wrote papers. 'I considered it to be very important to start giving papers so that we could talk about cochlear implants although without data, which was still being collected, it could be embarrassing. I would just pop up at conferences all over the place and thank God I had the freedom to do that, and just ask questions as an opportunity to talk about multi-channel cochlear implants and the Melbourne device.'

Mecklenburg and Brimacombe were always there for the first programming of a patient. They trained every clinician who programmed any patient in the USA and slowly built up a good team of audiologists. Mecklenburg flew to wherever there was a problem and phoned Jim Patrick if any device wasn't working 'to analyse various strategies to make the technology work. Jim flew over for some of these cases and so this is how wonderful the service was'. Nucleus offered the service at no cost to the patient and would go anywhere that was needed, no matter how many hours were required. Replacement units would arrive special delivery with no expense spared.

The Cochlear team was very professional, very confident and very fast responders. This kind of service made the chief competitor look very sluggish and slow. It also proved to US specialists that there wasn't anything to worry about if the device weren't made in the USA.

The team was very strict about the protocol at every stage of the process to ensure that FDA approval was not held up due to unreliable data. FDA approval was recognised as critical in the 1979 market survey, since 'the United States is likely to be the first major market for cochlear implants'. The market survey team first met FDA officials in September 1979, and even at that early stage the team impressed upon Clark the need for his documentation and trials to meet FDA requirements. Regulatory approval was a team effort involving multiple trips to Washington over several years, as well as the use of local advisers.

Just as the technological development of the implant owed much to the existing resources of the Nucleus Group, the parent company was also vital when it came to preparing the groundwork for regulatory approval. The Nucleus Group's association with US corporate lawyer Bill Nealon, who had extensive experience in US regulatory matters, provided knowledgeable assistance to Cochlear Corporation. The pre-market approval application submitted in 1984 ran to 3000 pages and involved meticulous preparation; as Hirshorn later explained, 'Some documents were even rewritten to correct the subtle differences between Australian and American English'. At the FDA panel hearing for the Nucleus System in 1985, one of the panel members commented that he had never seen such high-quality clinical data – a testimonial to the excellence with which the study was managed.

In early 1985 the findings and histories of 87 patients in three continents (USA, Europe and Australia) were analysed and presented to the FDA. In October 1985, the FDA approved the use of the Nucleus implant in adults who had hearing before going deaf. The Nucleus device was the first multi-electrode cochlear implant to be approved as safe and effective for clinical use, by any health regulator.

CHAPTER 8

A global market beckoned: Ron West, Monika Lehnhardt and Sue Roberts

In December 1984, Ron West was recruited as CEO of Nucleus' US subsidiary, Cochlear Corporation. Mike Hirshorn was very careful in his choice. In line with company strategy, his perception was that the subsidiary needed someone who understood the medical professional culture and could relate to the technology, not just focus on sales. West had been at Johnson & Johnson, where he worked for the ultrasound section of its cardiovascular business. He was interested in running a business but at Johnson & Johnson Ultrasound his only opportunity to do so was on the east coast, where he didn't want to go. He had decided to stay in Denver and do some consulting work while looking for an opportunity to run a business. In late July 1984, he was contacted by a recruiter for the Cochlear Corp CEO position. As part of the interview Hirshorn asked West to draw a heart. West said, 'I knew a little bit about cardiology so when he asked me to draw a heart, I thought that was fair. The interview went pretty well but I didn't think much about it. Cochlear was a start-up company and I wasn't sure I was really interested in all the issues that go on with a start-up company, especially fundraising.' Hirshorn was very thorough, checked all West's references and thought the best way to start was by getting to know each other better. So he hired West initially to do some consulting work. That strategy fitted with West's plans 'because that's what I was doing at that point in time anyway and I wasn't in a big hurry. He left me to help him with positioning the firm and some marketing work associated with the American Academy of Audiology conference that was to be conducted in the fall.' The conference was a success and West got the job.

As the new leader of the new subsidiary, West was charged with growing sales for the company to meet its current business plan objectives. Experienced in the US medical devices market, he was a crucial element in the business plan in that he provided a solution to its problem of not having business knowhow and connectivity in the US ENT market. However, a number of cultural and structural problems immediately came to the fore, making his acceptance of the role difficult.

Culturally, West had very little experience with firms outside the USA and he was sceptical whether the Cochlear Corp device could be dominant in the US marketplace. 'After all, Australia is not where you expect to find the best technology.' But he had experience with some other Nucleus technology and 'knew that they had some fairly sophisticated design tools'. On the other hand, he thought that the business plan numbers were staggering. 'They had the price going down 5% every year for the first 10 years and the demand going up dramatically and I just couldn't convince myself it was possible to move a business so fast.' He was also worried that the company, as a start-up, would be undercapitalised but was pacified in that the start-up was part of the Nucleus Group. Trainor refused to give him options and he had to renegotiate his contract to include a bonus scheme. When he tried to employ senior staff who needed to be paid US salaries, Nucleus did not initially see the need, and he had to employ less-qualified people. Also, the board was not always cooperative. It didn't always understand US requirements and at times West found board members to be quite hostile.

Several events, however, provided him with solutions. CEO David Money strongly believed that nationals knew their own market best and as long as they were producing results he did not interfere with their procedures. He had met West and thoroughly approved his appointment. West believed that 'under David's entire period we had a good working relationship and I think all the executives would really have struggled without his support'.

The pressure for profit had some interesting consequences. Mecklenburg's assistant, Judy Brimacombe, had a very memorable exchange with Money: she stood up in an internal company meeting and asked, 'David, what are your values?' Brimacombe was very distressed that Cochlear Corp was making money from people who suffered a hearing impairment. She only reluctantly accepted his argument that when a person is implanted they have the implant for life, and the only way that they can be assured of ongoing support is if Cochlear stayed in business. Money argued that the company's drive for profit was in the best interest of the patients, indeed was essential for them. This argument was the driving philosophy throughout the company's history and perhaps was one of the key strategies behind its current success. Cochlear Corp was in the business of giving hearing to people who were deaf. Once implanted, those people stayed in the company's care for life and to ensure that care was available the company had to stay in business. It was also Money's rationale for buying competitors that went out of business – his company took on their liabilities so that the industry would remain viable. However, his exchange with the audiologist clearly demonstrated the difficulty of balancing different value systems in the biotechnology industry and showed why it is critical to change leadership from the scientific to the commercial at an early phase of the company's growth process.

Another beneficial factor for the US team was that 3M had been in the market for a year, so the Cochlear team was not challenged with the problems of being a first entrant with a new technology. West and Brimacombe were the first Cochlear US sales team and visited all the clinics working with the 3M device because these people 'at least knew what the heck we were talking about'. Brimacombe developed a video showing how the patient received speech recognition from their device and this proved to be very effective. The first sale created great excitement and produced desperately needed revenue.

Rae Reynolds was hired by West in late 1985 to develop a market for Cochlear implants in the USA. She was concerned that, although the company had received FDA approval for adult implants and was running classes for surgeons, there 'weren't any people volunteering for implants and the doctors were saying they would love to do the surgery but had no idea where to find the deaf people'. Reynolds saw two obstacles to meeting the budget targets that the Australian head office had set. The first was that they had no customers and the second was that there was a major competitor – the House device – that was sold through a highly respected US corporate giant, 3M, with a wonderful reputation. ENT surgeons gave their loyalty to House. House also made sure that he was at all the surgeons' meetings promoting his device. However, his single-channel device was not as effective as the Cochlear multi-channel device and patients who had been implanted with the 3M device were not getting speech recognition and thus were not recommending that device to others. Furthermore, surgeons and audiologists did not understand that there was a significant difference between the two products and were reluctant to recommend either of them.

The solution was multi-tiered. First, West and his team expanded the work begun by Mecklenburg to educate additional surgeons and clinicians. They soon found a number of surgeons who were eager to promote their careers and do ground-breaking surgery. Although they knew and respected House, these surgeons saw an opportunity to do better with the implant that provided speech recognition. The trick was to identify those surgeons and to provide them with training and support. Cochlear Corp expanded its educational programs to audiologists, so they could appreciate the benefits of the Cochlear system and begin to recommend it. It was also very clear early in the process that medical insurance companies would have to be convinced of the benefits, in both the government Medicare system and the private systems, to reimburse patients who had received the implant. This was difficult. As with any new technology, until the agencies were educated about and agreed that there was a difference, the Melbourne implant was considered only a hearing aid. Insurers had written exclusions in their policies for hearing aids. To further complicate the matter, when the government did finally start to reimburse implants it was at a very low level. Doctors and hospitals were not covering their costs and thus were excluding Medicare patients from surgery. The problem was quite tricky in that many of the hospitals did not know just how much they were losing. If the Cochlear team were to advertise these facts in attempting to get government support, they would potentially lose that hospital market. The first major problem for the new subsidiary, therefore, was how to stimulate the market to generate more surgery and make more people aware of the fact that the device was potentially beneficial to them, while keeping doctors, hospitals and government agencies on side. The relationship-building was relentless, but the new team were just as driven and passionate as their Australian colleagues in Sydney and Melbourne.

It was obvious that Cochlear Corp should begin to market to the deaf community, but original strategies were required. Organisations of the deaf were the first to be approached. Public relations campaigns were generated, with newspaper advertisements announcing forums to showcase studies of people who had benefited from the device. A hotline was established to explain the device to the public. Advertisements were placed in audiology magazines, drawing distinctions about why this device was an improvement on the single-channel device. The company was the first to promote its device direct to consumers, but that brought its own problems.

Reynolds was astonished to find that 'the deaf community was against us'. The Cochlear team soon learnt that they had a formidable history to overcome. Prior to the 18th century, it was commonly supposed that congenitally deaf children were mute because they were stupid. Congenitally deaf people were treated as imbeciles and as a source of ridicule. However, a French priest, the Abbé de l'Epeé, devised an effective sign language that enabled deaf children to communicate. He demonstrated that deaf children had the same level of intelligence as their hearing peers. The Abbé broke the chains from the deaf, giving them self-esteem and allowing them to enjoy a new sense of freedom. They were not going to give this up easily.

The deaf disliked attempts to make them speak like hearing people. They preferred their own identity as Deaf people and insisted on spelling the word 'deaf' with a capital D. There was a whole industry and economic basis that supported this philosophy. There were sign language interpreters and teachers of the deaf and administrators of deaf institutions, and Cochlear was undermining their whole economic potential. But it wasn't till Cochlear received approval to implant the device into children that it really got ugly. These people attended forums and were very vocal in their attack on the device. Reynolds laments that many of the arguments over an implant versus sign language continue today even though the technology has been much improved and the benefits have been accepted to the point where not only the profoundly deaf but also the severely hearing-impaired are receiving implants.

Problems for West were further exacerbated by the Australian head office's lack of understanding of the US environment. For instance, Reynolds felt that the people in Australia were quite foolish in not providing any funds to lobby government bodies. 'It is just one of those things that you have to do to get attention is to be politically active. One of our major competitors had a couple of product recalls but these were not at all widely publicised or as devastating as they could have been without the connections that the company had in Washington.' Money saw this issue as a problem of opportunity cost. The cost of lobbying the US government would reduce funding in other areas of the business such as R&D, and was therefore not an option in his opinion.

Production problems were also an issue. The patient would be ready, surgery was scheduled but there would be no delivery of product. Sales reps would be sent out to borrow a back-up implant from somebody else so that the scheduled patient could have an implant – very embarrassing. Later, when approval had been received for children to be implanted, the busiest time for child implants was during the Christmas break – when the Australian office shut down for three weeks. 'We would have parents screaming down the phone because they had carefully rearranged their lives so that their child could get an implant during this brief window and the Australians were going on vacation. We were just going nuts.'

In addition, West worried that the Australians just did not understand the US market in terms of cosmetics. The product was initially produced only in a beige colour, which was fine if the patient were white. Being manufactured in Australia, which until the 1960s had adhered to a White Australia policy on immigration, there was no perceived problem, but implant colour was a real issue in the multicultural USA. West was frustrated that he had no control over even such decisions as small cosmetic changes to the device. Additional problems noted by the US team included the inability of the Australians to see the need for an extension of products such as their competitors had established, and the acquisition of groups that could extend their market. The major advantage for the company was always the superiority of the product. A further competitive advantage was the ever-present dedication and solutions-driven focus of its staff, although a focus-driven team poses its own challenges as the firm extends its operations.

West respected that Mecklenburg had been very strict about protocol to ensure successful FDA approval, and initially 'that kind of control can be justified because the study has to be done according to the protocol. We had a very interesting study as a result of Dianne's commitment and her control orientation but once we got through the clinical trial that kind of orientation became difficult to manage as we tried to put commercial systems in place and build up customer relationships.' Mecklenburg was used to running around the country and trouble-shooting, but

West needed her in the office in Denver. Mecklenburg didn't want to go to Denver. It was a difficult transition for the company. Hirshorn also had difficulty in letting go. West gave Hirshorn three going-away parties before he finally moved onto his next assignment, setting up a European subsidiary. West understood that 'Mike found it difficult to let go of what he had so brilliantly started', but there can only be one CEO and having put the US operation in place it was time for him to go.

• • •

In 1984 Graeme Clark phoned Sue Roberts, a recent audiology graduate, and said, 'We are now going to start working with younger patients on the implant program and I will need a qualified audiologist and speech pathologist. You are the only one I know with both these qualifications. Come and work with us and we will pay you about half of what you are earning now. So would you like the job?' It is a testament to Clark's ability to inspire people that Roberts accepted the offer, although never quite sure why she had done so. She started working in the department of audiology at the University of Melbourne (UOM) with Richard Dowell, Peter Busby and Peter Seligman. She programmed the speech processors and worked on speech production with the first teenagers implanted with the Nucleus device. Her job was interesting and she worked with a motivated, fun-loving team for two years. She loved the work but, when her husband was transferred to London, it looked like her career in the cochlear implant industry would come to an abrupt end.

Roberts met Money by chance in the hallway at UOM and asked about Cochlear in London. Money was not keen on her joining Cochlear – it would be a sales job, and what do audiologists know about that? But he relented and told her, 'There is this guy Mike Hirshorn in London so give him a call when you get there but I am not sure what he can do for you.' In the meantime, Seligman had already contacted Hirshorn, telling him that Roberts had been working with the UOM team on implants for a couple of years and encouraging him to employ her when she arrived in London.

On a freezing April day, Roberts called on Hirshorn at his home in London and said, 'Hi. I am Sue Roberts and I am hoping you can give me a job.' Hirshorn asked how many languages she spoke. 'Just English', she replied. That was not a good start in Europe. So he asked, 'What skills can you offer me?' She had a better answer this time. 'Well, I worked with Graeme Clark for the last couple of years and I worked with the first few kids that have been implanted so maybe I can help you sell the implants in the UK.' 'I am going to Venice tomorrow, do you want to come?' Hirshorn asked. Roberts immediately agreed, thinking, 'Oh dear. What have I done now?' She rang her husband of two months and said, 'I am going to Venice tomorrow with this bloke that I have just met from Cochlear. Are you OK with that?'

They arrived at the meeting next day in St Mark's Square, San Giovanni to a huge sea of male ENT surgeons. Hirshorn nudged her, saying, 'You have to ask Bill House a question, you have to show me that this trip was worth it.' Determined to get her job, she stood up and said, 'Hi. I am Sue Roberts and I am working for Cochlear. I have been working for the last two years with kids implanted with multi-channel devices in Australia.' She had their attention immediately because this was so new. As Roberts began to answer questions Hirshorn knew that she had the courage and intelligence to do the job, and decided to give her some work.

Ready for work, Roberts turned up at the Telectronics London office in Regent's Park but it was apparent that Telectronics really didn't want the Cochlear team there. Hirshorn and Roberts were given one very small corner of the office, but nothing else. Not even a chair. Roberts sat on a box for the first three months, sharing half a desk with Hirshorn. Her first job was to call on all Hirshorn's European contacts to find out how many implants they had done and what types of implants they were. She found that there were 37 different types of implants in Europe at that stage. There were single-channel implants, a two-channel, a four-channel and an eight-channel implant. There were lots of different cochlear implants but they were mainly prototypes. There were Austrian, English, French and even Spanish implants, all different. Roberts gathered the numbers and divided the market by percentages. Only a tiny percentage of the market was taken up by multi-channel implant devices where the electrode was inserted into the cochlea, apparently because most people didn't really believe a multi-channel device would provide speech recognition. It was also assumed that putting an electrode into the cochlea would damage any remaining hearing. They would have to make sure that they could demonstrate Clark's research that emphasised the device didn't damage the cochlea and truly provided speech recognition. The critical point to communicate was that the device works and it lasts a lifetime, therefore adding value to a profoundly deaf person's life.

The competitors didn't give up easily and there was a huge difference between the Australian price of $10 000 and the local price of $1000. At one conference Graham Fraser, an English ENT surgeon, was demonstrating his own English device. He stood up, pointed to the Cochlear team and said, 'You can arrive at the Ritz in a Rolls Royce but you can get there just as quickly in a Mini Minor' and he showed his single-channel implant. Hirshorn and Roberts were not without wit and their immediate response was, 'You can arrive at the Ritz in a Mini Minor but you will get a much better reception if you arrive in a Rolls Royce.' The slogan was made into a flyer and used to promote the multi-channel device.

As in the USA, competitors looked down on the Cochlear team. 'These Colonials, what can they know?' The attempts to outmanoeuvre each other never stopped, with Fraser addressing conferences saying, 'You know you have to pay all this money for this silly nanny to run around after you.' Roberts, with her Australian good looks, immediately stood up and said, 'Hi. I am a Nucleus nanny from London.' An ENT surgeon stood up and said, 'Hi nanny, obviously the better product!' Fraser laughed and said, 'On this occasion, I have no response.' However, when Lord Ashley of Stoke became his patient, Fraser conceded that the Cochlear multi-channel implant would provide a better outcome than his own device. He rang the Cochlear team and said, 'We want to use your implant.' Roberts was in Spain when she received the call and despite the heat she shuddered because although the opportunity was exciting and probably the most fantastic thing that could happen, given the high standing of the would-be patient, it could also end in complete disaster. Her stomach was very tight.

The device didn't work. When Fraser rang Roberts two days later to give her the news she nearly dropped the phone. She told him not to panic and had another device delivered and reimplanted immediately. The second implant was a success and Lord Ashley became a real advocate for Cochlear implants. Fraser immediately increased his lobbying efforts. He was basically lobbying for his cheaper single-channel implant but in the process he was also helping the cochlear implant industry by increasing awareness of all the possibilities in the market. Due to his lobbying, Cochlear received a grant for 120 implants and joined Fraser in his lobbying efforts.

By 1988 they were implanting the multi-channel device in Manchester, England and in Kilmarnock and Ayreshire in Scotland. As the London office grew Hirshorn made a decision to establish the European head office in a country from where he could operate without taxes to distribute the implants. The CEO David Money agreed that the head office in Europe should be in a neutral country in continental Europe rather than in England. They were particularly concerned not to locate in France and Germany, both of which had their own systems and which evoked unnecessary emotional reactions. Switzerland seemed a logical choice as it was a small high-tech country with the advantage of lower taxes. Initially Money had investigated Zug, near Zürich, but Hirshorn eventually chose Basel which was judged to be the most central city at the 'three-countries corner' where Switzerland, Germany and France meet. Germany was obviously a major market due to the fact that the Cochlear team had managed to attract the most influential ENT surgeon in Europe, Professor Ernst Lehnhardt, onto the European board.

Before Cochlear had a presence in Europe, Money attended a symposium on cochlear implants in Erlangen, Germany, in 1982. There he gave an impromptu presentation on the Nucleus system, which was printed in the proceedings. He then met Dianne Mecklenburg and spent a further couple of weeks in Germany, cold-calling ENT surgeons from the phone book and arranging to visit them to increase the level of knowledge and interest in cochlear implants. Hirshorn also cold-called on ENT surgeons in Europe to make initial contacts in an effort to establish the business. In some cases, after making the appointment and taking a long, cold train ride he arrived to find a younger-than-expected man waiting for him. The surgeon he thought he had made an appointment with was no longer practising; the son had taken over the practice but was not interested in cochlear implants. At other times it was a little easier to reach surgeons by using the contacts that had been made earlier, specifically Lehnhardt who was operating in Hannover.

During his 1982 trip to Europe, Money had visited Lehnhardt and his engineer, Rolf Battmer, in Hannover. They asked him to speak about the Nucleus system before an audience from a local technical university that was developing its own system. His talk was very well received, with consequent growing interest in the UOM device in Europe. Lehnhardt had also met Hirshorn a few years earlier at a conference where Hirshorn had shown him a model of the device. This was at a time when Lehnhardt had been working with the Max-Planck Institute on developing its own cochlear implant in Germany. Lehnhardt and Battmer paid their own fares to Australia to see a demonstration of the prototype. Clark had met them at the airport in Melbourne. As he watched the sophisticated Lehnhardt stepping off the plane, unshaven and in a bad mood from the length of time he had spent on the plane, Clark thought, 'Oh dear. How are we going to impress these two worldly doctors?' He need not have worried. They were so impressed that they championed the UOM cochlear implant program in Hannover and convinced the Max-Planck Institute to stop work on its device, since Lehnhardt considered there was no need to 'reinvent the wheel'. It was Lehnhardt who wrote the first audiology textbook for Europe and enthusiastically converted German ENT surgeons to support the Australian cochlear implant. Having him as a champion in Europe was indeed a great coup. Whoever Hirshorn employed to lead the European division would need to work closely with the eminent professor.

Hirshorn advertised widely for the CEO role and eventually received an application from Monika Lange, who had been born in Vienna and had graduated from the University Alma Mater Rudolfina there. She had earned a PhD in philology, psychology and philosophy and spoke nine languages fluently. Her résumé said that she had held various positions in companies such as Schering (Berlin), Monsanto (Düsseldorf and Brussels) and Pharmacia (Freiburg). An appointment was organised and Hirshorn asked David Rigg, who was in charge of the Telectronics London office at the time, to assist with the interview.

Lange was poised, intelligent and confident and her CV indicated that she had a lot of experience working for Pharmacia. It was not directly in the ENT area but still in the medical industry, just a different aspect of it. Sitting on her box in the corner of the room, Roberts thought, 'Oh my gosh I am going to have an interesting time now. The woman even speaks nine languages.' Other suitable candidates had been located, but Lange was offered the job. Money highly approved the appointment.

But Lange was not immediately overly excited with the offer. Cochlear brought her to Australia to meet the head office people and she was not impressed. She sat in her room at the Artarmon Inn on the very busy Pacific Highway in the middle of Sydney suburbia and wondered what she was doing there. Having worked for major pharmaceutical companies in Europe, Lange was used to five-star hotels and very sophisticated people and facilities. Also, German society was very hierarchical, for instance people did not say 'Professor Ernst' but rather 'Herr Doctor Professor Lehnhardt'. In Australia it was so informal, unsophisticated and apparently lacking in structure that Lange decided, waiting in her suburban motel room for a taxi to take her to the airport, to turn the offer down. But then the phone rang: Jim Patrick had called to say that he was so glad she was joining them and what a terrific difference she would make to their efforts in Europe. That phone call changed Lange's mind. She went on to take over the London office and established Cochlear Europe in Basel in 1987.

Hirshorn returned to Australia, leaving Roberts and Lange to work together. The target budget for the year left them breathless but Lange was determined to achieve it. However, if West thought he had cultural problems in the USA, those were nothing to the differences about to take place in Cochlear Europe. There was a major cultural divide between the young Aussie who just wanted to get on with the job and be friendly, and the more formal Lange and her assistant Ulrike. Roberts felt like she was being hounded on a daily basis, but once she got over the cultural divide she began to understand why it had to be 'Herr Doctor Professor Lehnhardt'. Giving a person the wrong title was a major mistake and actually considered an insult – a real eye-opener for the young Australian. Roberts eventually also understood why Lange's purchase of red leather chairs and expensive desks for the Basel office was justified although Roberts' seat in the London office was a box. Money was apoplectic about the extravagance but Lange was adamant that if they were to have a presence in Europe they would need to be impressive.

It was not long before Ernst von Wallenberg joined them and all four focused on sales, training surgeons and clinicians. Given Mecklenburg's problems working with West's leadership, the company did not want to lose her and offered her a position in Cochlear Europe. The cultural divide slowly melted and, being focused on the same goals, the team eventually learnt to love each other. They were all intelligent and really good fun, which in the end was the real connection, and would strategise how they could win the European surgeons' hearts and minds. Lange was the one who figured out how to get around people and Roberts just tried to be friendly. Because of Lange's haughtiness and her Viennese attitude, people either loved her or disliked her. The Australian approach, on the other hand, reached the middle ground. Together, Lange and Roberts made a good team.

Roberts worked on increasing sales to the UK market as well as the Middle East and Scandinavian markets. The Middle East was a challenge for a woman. A female colleague who had previously worked for Hewlett Packard told a scary tale of having been arrested for prostitution when entering Saudi Arabia because she talked to a passenger in the immigration queue. Roberts managed to stay safe. Lange focused on the German ENT market, which was the biggest volume market. Germany and Switzerland gave the biggest unit sales. Eventually Cochlear Europe grew from two to 70 employees and opened additional offices in Hannover. Lange travelled extensively in Central and Eastern Europe and was responsible for 18 countries from Russia to the Baltic, Ukraine and Kazakhstan.

Hirshorn had hoped that Lange would work closely with Lehnhardt because he was such an important supporter in Europe. She certainly took her job seriously. One evening in Sydney when the whole overseas team had been brought together, Roberts was driving over the Harbour Bridge with a colleague when they suddenly saw Lange skipping hand in hand with Lehnhardt on the pedestrian walkway, her sandals in her hand. Roberts nearly crashed her car. The cover was blown, and Monika Lange soon became Monika Lehnhardt.

Despite close working relations, problems in Europe were similar to those in the USA. Head office in Australia was demanding ever-increasing sales figures and just didn't seem to understand that there was a very competitive market in Europe. Prices were being reduced by competitors at a frightening rate. As in the USA, sometimes Cochlear Europe would make a sale but there would be no product to deliver to the buyer. Not because the manufacturing teams in Sydney were inefficient, but because the system was very complex and difficult to manufacture.

Leo Port was in charge of manufacturing the external parts and there were multiple reasons why his team was not able to keep up with the demand in Europe and the USA. Only a small number of the components such as integrated circuits, capacitors and plastic parts that went into the devices were actually produced in Australia. Most came from overseas, and the Australian manufacture was dependent on a chain of people for supply and deliveries. The links in the chain had their own chains and deliveries were often held up. It was extraordinarily difficult to maintain a low but adequate inventory count. Constant development meant that having a big inventory was useless because products became obsolete very quickly. Port found himself having to go to the USA because of cable issues, to try and find a company that could manufacture cables for the speech processor. He had to go to Japan because of problems in the flexible circuit boards that went inside the ear implant. It was a ground-breaking industry and no one in Australia could supply most of their needs. It was a process of constant improvisation.

As in the USA, the deaf community in Europe staged campaigns against all forms of cochlear implants. In Birmingham, England protests were organised and deaf literature described a cochlear implant as a box with wires that surgeons put inside people's heads and that produced no value. Sometimes, the Cochlear team found patients with failed implants of competitor devices. For example, there were problems with the patients' skin and the percutaneous plugs used by some competitor devices, and some of the surgery hadn't been done in a very sensible way. Such problems gave the protesters more ammunition.

Perhaps one of the biggest demonstrations took place in a major ENT conference in Paris. The Deaf Society arrived and invaded the conference. They had brought whistles; as each speaker commenced their presentation, the protesters blew their whistles at the top of their lungs. Of course, the meeting couldn't go on. In France at that time anyone with a disability was allowed to demonstrate for that disability, and the police were not legally allowed to touch a disabled person. Each time the conference organisers tried to restart, the deaf community began blowing whistles again. An evening operatic performance had been organised in Notre Dame and it was assumed that the deaf community had left. No one imagined that they would buy tickets that cost several hundred francs, to listen to an opera that they could not hear. As delegates sat in hushed silence ready for the performance to begin, the assumption was proved wrong. Delegate after delegate stood up and noisily walked out, totally destroying the effect. It was a very strong demonstration and only one of many.

Despite the problems, the US and European divisions continued to make steady inroads into the cochlear market. In 1987, when the FDA approved implants for children, the market expanded substantially. As speech processors were improved, an additional market in updates began to grow.

The CEO, David Money, deserves credit for much of the initial company success in keeping the company on a growth path. His depth of experience in the design and manufacture of implants and his balanced approach to management issues earned him respect from the rest of the team and his Nucleus bosses. When they were shocked by their first, inevitable implant failures, Money had a perspective that others lacked. He demonstrated that their low but finite failure incidence was to be expected. At the same time he initiated the current practice that every failure be thoroughly analysed to identify the cause of failure, and that the knowledge be used to improve future designs. Cochlear's excellent implant reliability record is due in part to this.

Trainor's confidence in the success of the corporation was vindicated by the fact that by 1987 Nucleus' annual report could state that Cochlear was now well established as the market leader worldwide in cochlear implants, a position which it has maintained ever since. In 1989 3M admitted defeat and exited the industry. Cochlear purchased the 3M implant technology in a move to reassure patients and maintain confidence in the fledgling industry.

CHAPTER 9.

Without surgeons it was just clever engineering: Bill Gibson

With the completion of the commercial design and manufacture of the implantable device, it was time to change the focus from engineering to the patient. ENT surgeons in Australia and around the world were key to the connection. They championed the promotion of the device and struggled to garner support for the acceptance of a multi-channel cochlear implant that could give speech recognition to the profoundly deaf.

As in other parts of the world, there was opposition from the Deaf community. In Australia attempts were still being made to teach deaf children to speak but there were shifting ideas on the most appropriate thing to do. Lip-reading alone was not sufficient as only 30% of words can be lip-read. The lip-reader must use these words as clues to the meaning of the conversation. It is like doing a constant crossword puzzle, something that many cannot do. So acoustic devices were developed to aid those with hearing loss. Although hearing aids improved over the years, they could only amplify residual hearing. They could not provide sufficient amplification for the profoundly deaf. Even with powerful hearing aids, the higher frequencies typically can't be heard. A deaf person hears vowel sounds but not the consonants. For example, if someone says, 'She goes shopping' the deaf person hears, 'He go hoppin', copies the sounds and speaks with those sounds, thus listeners can become confused. An auditory oral approach was popularised in the 1950s and 1960s. Children were forced to sit on their hands to prevent them signing. They were taught to use lip-reading and tactile clues, to learn to speak. It was a disaster. With few exceptions, for example if a parent were prepared to spend countless hours working with their child, most children developed only poor speech which could not be understood.

121

In Australia in the 1970s and 1980s, it became politically correct again to allow deaf children to use sign language. As it was realised that most deaf children who only signed had very poor reading and writing skills, a method called Total Communication was developed. The children had to use signed English in which every word is signed in grammatical context. This is very slow and cumbersome. The deaf children were also expected to learn some speech using hearing aids. When they left school they usually threw away their hearing aids and enjoyed using fluent sign languages such as Auslan (Australian Sign Language).

Professor William Gibson had always been interesting in the ear and its workings. He was born in a town in Devon, England and trained in London to become an ear, nose and throat surgeon. He became interested in cochlear implants through a program called Project Ear, which promoted the concept of cochlear implants. He was further impressed in 1982 when he met Graeme Clark at the Royal Society of Medicine and they discussed Clark's project in Melbourne.

Gibson had an identical twin who had married an Australian woman and, during a visit to Australia, Gibson and his family decided that it wouldn't be a bad place to live. When he saw an advertisement for the position of Head of ENT Department at the University of Sydney, he applied immediately. He got the job and emigrated to Australia with his family in 1983.

This was good timing for an ENT surgeon interested in electrophysiology. Nucleus had just completed commercial development of the University of Melbourne (UOM) prototype and six patients were in the process of being implanted, with amazing success. Although it was still two years before FDA approval would be granted, Gibson was approached by Mike Hirshorn, who welcomed him to Sydney and offered to provide two free Nucleus implants to begin the cochlear implant program in Royal Prince Alfred Hospital, the University of Sydney teaching hospital. This was an excellent beginning for a new Head of Department. Each implant normally cost $10 000 so the offer was equivalent to $20 000, and Gibson was very keen to get involved in such ground-breaking development. But he needed to do some political manoeuvring. The University of Sydney was very conservative and Clark was being criticised by the elder statesmen of ENT surgeons, who considered the research was futile. Gibson was careful to seek permission from his department before he dared to go ahead. A well-connected colleague, Barrie Scrivener, was his greatest supporter and lobbied to help Gibson get the project started.

As an ENT surgeon, Gibson belonged to the Toynbee Club. The club met each year, alternating between the Melbourne Club and the Australian Club in Sydney, for a black-tie dinner. Late in 1983, Gibson was asked to give the dinner speech on his intentions, as a new professor at the University of Sydney, for the progress of the ENT department. Gibson outlined several projects and spoke about his intention to commence using Clark's cochlear implant, which was now commercially available. He had no idea of the storm of criticism this would produce. Cochlear had provided the implants but encouraged Gibson to find further financial assistance from the University of Sydney to carry out the program. Funding was not forthcoming, but Scrivener again saved the day. Scrivener sat on the board of the School for the Deaf and Blind Children and, with his encouragement, the school supported Gibson with financial assistance to carry on the implant program.

Financial support for cochlear programs has always been critical even if the device itself is given free. Although the cochlear implant is a piece of implantable electronics, as a prosthesis, it is much more than that. There is a surgical procedure and much work was done by Clark and his team to refine implantation techniques. The whole implant system includes an externally worn sound processor, or speech processor as it was initially called. Crucial to a successful outcome is the audiology and programming of the external device.

The audiologist's job starts well before implantation. Patient selection is key to a good outcome. The first step is a range of hearing tests. It is important not to implant a person who could be better fitted with a hearing aid. It is equally important not to implant when there is no chance of a successful outcome. The hearing tests are accompanied by CT scans or MRIs. The decisions on whether to implant and if so, in which ear, are generally made by a panel including a number of audiologists and surgeons. The pros and cons of the case and the specific ear are discussed in detail in light of the audiological tests, the potential implantee's medical condition, aetiology, family support, linguistic capabilities, access to clinic etc. If it is appropriate to go ahead the patient is offered the procedure. The patient and family are counselled to avoid unrealistic expectations.

Once a decision has been made and the surgery has been carried out there is usually a short period of recuperation, generally a few days to a few weeks. The 'switch on' occurs after a post-operation medical examination, a visit to the audiology clinic and the use of some specialised hardware. The clinic has a computer interface and software to carry out the required tests and program the information into the sound processor. Each cochlear implant and each sound processor must be compatible to allow clinicians to program the people who have just been implanted.

Additional to the programming aspects of the software, the implant is capable of providing feedback on its operation. Electrode characteristics, neural responses and diagnostic information are returned via the software to the audiologist. The results are tabulated and graphed. On the big day, the clinician, usually an audiologist but in some countries an acoustician, surgeon, engineer, nurse or technician, sits in a room with the patient and usually some close family members. Again, everyone is cautioned against unrealistic expectations.

The beginning is slow. The sound processor is placed on the patient's ear and connected to the programming interface, which is connected to the computer. The patient's coil is put in place behind the ear and the magnet is adjusted to the right strength. Too tight, and it can cause skin damage or necrosis. Too weak, and it will annoyingly fall off.

The patient is given instructions by lip-reading, written notes or gestures. 'Tap with the pen when you hear a sound.' The stimuli are sent to the implant and gradually increased in level. Using the software, the clinician measures the threshold level of hearing for each electrode or group of electrodes. 'Now tap when the sound you hear is loud but comfortable.' There are 22 electrodes, thus measuring the threshold and comfortable level of each electrode involves 44 judgments. The clinician then sets the program to sweep through a small number of electrodes at a time. 'Tell me if they are the same loudness. Which ones were louder? Which were softer?' Adjustments are made. So far the patient has heard nothing but beeps and buzzes. The clinician is now in a position to select a sound-coding strategy in which the stimulation rate for the electrical pulses and the number of electrodes is set. Several other choices are made. If all is well, the clinician will usually choose the current default parameters. The moment of truth comes. The patient is counselled, 'I'm going to switch it on now.' A big green button is clicked on the screen and the system goes 'live'. The reactions are many and varied. Sometimes tears, surprise, disappointment, confusion. The clinician speaks, the family member speaks. 'Hello. Can you hear me? How does my voice sound?' Some patients can start to make use of the strange sound immediately. Some are bemused. Some are overwhelmed with emotion.

Once the initial reaction has passed, the clinician makes adjustments. Was speech too loud, too soft? Many recipients with a progressive hearing loss have not heard anything high-pitched for years and find the new sound unfamiliar and often unpleasant at first, although it does contain much useful information. The re-learning process begins.

After some adjustments a program or map, as it is called, is loaded into the processor. Sometimes a number of maps are loaded for the patient to try out. The patient and family are instructed on the use of the processor and its settings. The patient is encouraged to try these out in as many situations as possible. An appointment is made for another visit in a week or so. The intervals between visits gradually increase – monthly, six-monthly, annually – and the visits are often combined with a quick surgical check-up.

When the patient is a child or an infant, the clinician's job is much harder. Neural response telemetry (NRT) indicates when nerve firing is first detected. Unfortunately, the correspondence with the perceptual experience is not always very close and compensation for the loudness difference or tilt of the profile of responses has to be made. Clinicians dealing with babies develop great skill in looking at the child's responses and eye blinks, head turns and expressions.

Aside from the issues of hearing, speech production may need attention. Those who have missed out on the crucial periods of speech development usually speak with distinctive 'deaf speech', often unintelligible to those who are unfamiliar with it. Much hard work on the part of patients and speech pathologists is required to unlearn this deaf speech.

As with any medical intervention, things don't always work out the way people hope or expect. Every patient is different. With surgery as complex as that of a cochlear implant, plus the variability of the cochlea and the variability of aetiology, a wide range of outcomes is possible. Clinics sometimes need help and troubleshooting by telephone and visits from travelling Cochlear staff.

Although the process is complex, the results of Gibson's first implants were outstanding and both recipients were able to use the cochlear implant to hear speech without using lip-reading. Gibson filmed a telephone conversation with one recipient and cheekily showed it to the senior ENT surgeons at the next Toynbee meeting, in 1984. They were not amused. He smiled when not a single question was asked after his speech and the meeting briskly passed to the next item on the agenda.

For Gibson, as for everyone connected with the multi-channel cochlear implant project, money was always scarce in the early days and each patient had to fully fund their own implant. The Vice Chancellor of the University of Sydney, Professor John Ward, helped Gibson to establish the EAR Foundation at the university in an effort to promote the concept. Gibson was desperately keen to perform the surgery on congenitally deaf children but he soon discovered that not only the Deaf community but the professional establishment was opposed to the idea. Gibson was told about all the failures of auditory oral teaching and that total communication was the best option for deaf children.

Professor John Yu had set up the Children's Hospital in Sydney and used his artistic skills to create a very colourful and welcoming place. He was very astute at political negotiation and suggested that Gibson bring all the different professional groups together, to create an atmosphere of collaboration that would bring ownership of the program to all those who would be involved and who currently might be antagonistic to the idea. The Profound Deafness Study Group was established for this purpose and Gibson met all the professionals each month to discuss the best way of beginning a children's cochlear implant program. It was soon obvious to him, however, that the group's main task was not to promote the idea but to dissuade him from hasty action. The hospital had just produced a film called 'Talking Hands', which showed parents how to sign to their deaf children. The group was dominated by people who strongly believed, in the fashion of the day, that deaf children should sign. It became apparent very early that they were appalled by the idea that Gibson was going to try to give deaf children hearing. They said that the hearing would be no good and would leave the child in no man's land, and did everything they could to slow the progress of the implant project.

In 1987 Gibson performed his first implants on young children, in gross contradiction to the wishes of the Profound Deafness Study Group. The first three children had been deafened by meningitis. One was a young girl called Holly, whose father was a fisherman working on the Hawkesbury River. The family lived in a bay which could only be reached by boat. Holly went suddenly deaf when she was about three and a half and started to lose her speech because of her complete deafness. She had formerly played with a little boy, named Jolly, next door but when she went deaf she wouldn't go near Jolly any more.

Gibson saw her for an unrelated reason and suggested an implant but Holly was not quite five years old and no one at that time had done implant surgery on a child so young. The youngest recipient was a seven-and-a-half year old who had been operated on by Clark. Gibson was asked how he knew the implant would work. Members of the deaf community heard about the proposed operation and were horrified. One of the community leaders went to see the parents and said that the surgery hadn't been done before on such a young child, it was very strange and it wouldn't work. The leader offered Holly a place in Chatswood Primary School's Opportunity D (OD) unit, where she could learn to sign. 'What did the parents want?' the community leader asked. 'Some kind of miracle?'

Holly's parents decided, however, that she would have the implant. The child went from strength to strength. She got her voice back quite quickly once she could hear again. She came second in her regular class at Chatswood Primary, went to the University of Sydney and eventually graduated with first-class Honours in Law. But one of the first things she did when she got her hearing back was to begin playing with Jolly again. Her mother always thought, 'That miracle? I think we got it.'

The first congenitally deaf child to be operated on was Pia Jeffery. Her half-sister Kitty was not deaf but their mother carried the gene, as did Pia's father, resulting in Pia being born profoundly deaf. Pia's reaction to her switch-on was enchanting. In 1992, the back cover of the telephone directory delivered to every home in the city showed a full-page photo of Pia having her device switched on. Her expression of amazement and joy told a wonderful story that encouraged other people to approach Cochlear. Yet despit the successful surgery and results, Gibson received a barrage of mail condemning his actions and as a consequence Yu disbanded the Profound Deafness Study Group.

The exposure did, however, increase awareness in Sydney of the effectiveness of the device and was excellent from the fundraising viewpoint. Peter Anderson, the NSW Minister of Health, gave the Royal Prince Alfred Hospital funding to implant 10 adults each year. The Yenebis family donated money to the Children's Hospital at Camperdown for a cochlear implant centre, which Yu agreed to build on the third floor of Wade House. Together with research fellow Christopher Game and engineer Halit Sanli, the centre was designed for cochlear implant use.

However, overwhelming opposition to the centre continued to come from within the hospital, from the audiologists, paediatricians and social workers. Yu decided, after it had been completed, that the new space would be used for audiology instead of a cochlear implant centre. The Yenebis family withdrew its donation. The hospital administration was not pleased, but Yu stood firm and Gibson had to look elsewhere to establish his cochlear centre.

New South Wales at this time had only one state school teaching deaf children orally – Chatswood Primary School, which had a special deaf unit run by Maggie Loaney and Sylvia Romanik. The other oral institutions were the Shepherd Centre and St Gabriel's School. All were under political pressure to support Deaf culture and teach the children to sign.

There were several deaf pupils at Chatswood Primary, and the small teaching team was given a cupboard outside a classroom in which to keep their apparatus. During the lunch hour, Loaney and Romanik were allowed to use a classroom to program and teach the children. Peter Collins was NSW Minister for Health at the time. He visited Chatswood Primary and gave the team a grant to staff the house in nearby Anderson St that had been rented by Gibson, and to provide devices and follow-up services for 10 children each year.

Two major difficulties occurred. The senior teacher of the deaf decided to take control of the program and stop increasing the number of implants, and instead research in detail the children already implanted. After a power struggle, Gibson persuaded her to resign and take a non-clinical research role. About a month later he was summoned to Yu's office for a discussion, as the teacher claimed that she had been wrongly dismissed and her job description had been changed illegally. Her claim was overruled after an inquiry and she resigned from the program. Two months later, two auditors visited Gibson's office and he found that he had been accused of misappropriating EAR Foundation funds. A major committee of inquiry was set up under Professor James McLeod and for four months Gibson was quizzed on everything he had done. The committee checked every dollar that had been spent. Gibson felt fairly secure since he had not claimed even a bus fare from the EAR Foundation, but he knew that if he had inadvertently made an error he would certainly lose his job and would probably have to return to England. After several stressful months, it was determined that every dollar had been properly spent. The inquiry even found some funds which had been redirected to another university department; the funds were returned to the EAR Foundation.

Another crisis was that Gibson was accused of running a brothel in Anderson St. The neighbours had seen young women going to and from the house, and had jumped to the wrong conclusion. Gregory Bartels, Mayor of Willoughby at the time, assisted Gibson through the council meeting and explained that Gibson had to gain proper council approval for the activities in the future. It was not long, however, before the house in Anderson St became too small. Bartels found a suitable house in Narrabeen, a northern beaches suburb of Sydney, and made sure that all appropriate council approvals were received. It wasn't long before the second house also became too small. Staff numbers had increased to eight and using one of the bathrooms as a temporary office wasn't really suitable. Gibson managed to get the Variety Club of Australia to commit to building a centre in the grounds of Concord Hospital in Sydney's inner west.

The chairman of Gibson's group, Bert Healy, was a retired architect. He designed a suitable centre, but at the last moment he and Gibson were summoned to the office of Concord Hospital CEO Professor Diana Horvath, where Deputy CEO Michael Wallace told them it had been decided that Concord Hospital grounds were unsuitable for such a venture. It was obviously a political decision because at the time there was an attempt to close Concord Hospital. Healy was very disappointed and in frustration resigned from his role as chairman.

In 1996 two significant events occurred. The group received a grant from the NSW Health Department that allowed use of part of the Gladesville Hospital, a disused mental hospital, and Christopher Rehn was appointed General Manager of the group. Rehn provided much-needed management skills and it has been said that much of the group's progress in those years was due to his abilities. Gibson's wife Alexandra and Doug Herridge spent countless hours over several weeks decorating and refurbishing the bleak old rooms at Gladesville to become a cochlear implant centre, which was officially opened by then NSW Minister for Health, Andrew Refshauge. Finally, the group had a home for children's cochlear implants. Then the Royal Prince Alfred cochlear implant centre for adults, in the basement of the hospital's residency building, became homeless due to redevelopment; after some persuasion Gibson was able to move that program to the Gladesville site. For a while the children's and adults' programs remained separate, but they finally merged to become the Sydney Cochlear Implant Centre (SCIC). By 1998 the centre had about 500 recipients of cochlear implants.

Gibson had never imagined how rapidly everything would progress – by 2010 there were over 2000 recipients. The success of the cochlear implant is apparent. It is accepted that the congenitally deaf children who receive a cochlear implant at an early age will learn to communicate so well using speech alone that they can be educated in mainstream schools. In NSW, signed English has been totally abandoned for younger children. Every school in NSW teaches the children orally, except one at North Rocks which offers Auslan. This is mainly for the children born to Deaf parents, although many Deaf parents now ask for their deaf children to receive a cochlear implant. Many more deafened adults also request cochlear implants so they can return to work, socialise and enjoy family life. The oldest recipient is 93 years old.

Much has changed from the early days of struggle. Today, SCIC at Gladesville has 40 staff members, including four surgeons. Another SCIC has been established in Newcastle, only two hours drive from Sydney, with eight staff members and four surgeons. There is an SCIC in Canberra, with three staff members and one surgeon.

SCIC recently opened another centre in Gosford on the NSW Central Coast. It is also associated with a very special centre in Bronte, the Matilda Rose Centre, which caters for children with other significant disabilities. SCIC outreaches to every major town in NSW and to Darwin, and offers services to nearby developing countries.

Professor Bill Gibson has every right to be proud of the group's development. Every NSW state government, whether Labor or Liberal, has supported his vision and the current government is no exception. However, it has been a rough road despite the government support. Gibson was subject to challenges similar to those Clark faced when he was criticised for his research and his very position at the UOM was under threat. This appears to be the burden that faces any such ground-breaking activity but, without the strength and courage of surgeons such as Clark and Gibson, where would the deaf people be?

CHAPTER 10

The entrepreneur bids adieu: Paul Trainor

Nanette Trainor was an intelligent, sophisticated woman. She enthusiastically supported her husband's ambition of developing his own global medical devices company in Australia and didn't argue when he wanted to sell their home to raise capital to fund that vision. She packed their belongings and moved the family to a rented home by the railway tracks, leaving their home in a prestigious neighborhood in the lower north shore suburb of Mosman. She left her wide social circle. She stood by her man and fulfilled all the home duties involved in raising three beautiful boys. But it was difficult. Very difficult. Even though articles in magazines such as the *Australian Women's Weekly* encouraged women to support their husbands, it was hard to cope when there were dinners that had been cooked but that no one turned up to eat. Sometimes, she finished the wine on her own. There were many empty nights when she needed help to get to sleep. Tragically, on 6 September 1986 the Trainors' second son, Benedict, died in a boating accident, and dependence on assistance to get through the days and nights slowly crept up on Nan Trainor. On 11 February 1987, she just didn't wake up.

Paul Trainor was shattered, although he had known that all was not well. Nan had sometimes arrived at functions heavily made up and wearing sunglasses to hide bleary eyes, but Trainor had considered it to be a 'woman's problem' and thought that 'real men didn't ask questions'. He knew that he had not always been there for Nan, but building the company was an enormous job. It was full-on. There were times when a huge number of issues needed immediate attention. There were times when the share price fell to 25c and journalists delighted in calling him a 'one-hit wonder'.

He had to respond to such comments, so there was constant pressure. Handling a kaleidoscope of people from different backgrounds, nationalities and disciplines meant that Trainor had to use every ounce of his people-management skills to meld this disparate group into effective working teams. The pressure of choosing the right people was never-ending. It was very time-consuming and he had to be abroad a lot of the time. His job could not be done sitting in an office in Sydney. He had to be in the USA, he had to be in Europe and Japan – wherever he was required. He knew that he was often exhausted when he did get home, but that was business and wives were meant to understand.

The family had moved from the house next to the railway tracks. Within four years of leaving Mosman they were living in a beautiful location in Hunter's Hill and, until Ben's tragic death, Trainor had thought that family life was working okay – barring the usual teenage problems. The boys, Dominic, Benedict and Matthew, were well provided for and Nan ensured that all their friends were welcome and very well fed. Matt was not interested in the business but Dom and Ben had met people from different industries and countries who were part of Trainor's 'other' family. This external family of dedicated colleagues and co-workers in Nucleus had been essential in helping to create and sustain his enormous venture. His plans and dreams may never have been fulfilled without their dedication, so Trainor considered them his second family and they filled most hours of his day. Until Ben's death, Trainor had been proud that he would be able to combine his two families through Ben, who had shown interest in and aptitude for becoming a potential successor. Ben had earned a Bachelor of Arts in Economics Law at Macquarie University and studied business management in Boston. He had also spent a year in the USA, learning the business. Now, in a space of five months, tragedy had twice undermined the direction of his hopes.

The two deaths knocked Trainor around badly, at a time when he was already concerned about Nucleus' future financial needs. He had been conscious that he had built the business as the controlling shareholder, which meant that he could do things that were adventurous or based on intuition and that he would never have managed to get past a typical board. As the controlling shareholder, Trainor had the freedom to follow his instincts and make a success of them but he knew that the business would constantly require more capital for its extensive R&D requirements and the never-ending need to keep ahead of competitors' existing products. Telectronics was developing a defibrillator product which was going to be the next big thing in pacemakers. The innovative device would use a dual chamber instead of a single chamber and would open up a new market for defibrillators, but it required a lot of additional R&D money. At the same time Cochlear was really expanding and needed additional funding. Between the two drivers, Nucleus needed a lot more money than it could secure from its current assets. The development of distribution markets into new areas would also involve capital, especially in the emerging technology companies that Trainor was building.

Given his style, there was no doubt that he would have found it very difficult to press on if he was not the controlling shareholder. He had no doubt that dilution of the existing ownership would leave Nucleus open to a hostile takeover. Having put so much into the business, Trainor didn't want to hold the business back and now, with the loss of his successor and his life partner, there appeared to be no option but to sell the company. He had already discussed the possibility with his family. Like his research, which was always planned five to 10 years in advance, there was a plan that looked five to 10 years ahead to when Trainor should exit. The family had considered how to handle it if he should die. Trainor discussed Nucleus with his two remaining sons and they agreed that selling it was the most appropriate strategy.

For six months Trainor secretly searched for a local company to carry on his work. He analysed Australian companies that were nationalistic, eventually selecting 10, which he studied and commissioned outside reports on. The list was whittled down to three. Trainor stipulated that the purchasing company had to have international flair and knowledge and be capable of exporting. It had to demonstrate an understanding of human behaviour that was fair and honest to staff. It also had to be willing to follow Trainor's principles of giving shares as well as remuneration to staff, which he believed would give the groups autonomy to continue into the 1990s. He was adamant that if the business had to be sold, it would be to an Australian group. 'Multi-nationals', he said, 'will pay us lip service and a lot of money, but they'll take our wealth away and 10 years from now our kids won't have jobs. They'll be making beds for foreign tourists.' Having made the decision, Trainor saw the sale simply as a baton change. He had worked to take Nucleus to a stage but he could not take it any further, so was willing to pass it on to an Australian company. But it wasn't easy to find a suitable company in Australia.

Trainor eventually decided that Pacific Dunlop was a very successful conglomerate and there was no reason why it couldn't make a success of Nucleus. It had made a success of tyres, it had made a success of cables and it had the capital to make a success of Nucleus. It was a public company on solid financial ground, giving it the financial strength to take Nucleus into the 1990s with the continuation of present growth. It had demonstrated keenness to move into new industries, so Trainor anticipated that it would protect the interests of his employees in a culture close to his own, and would promote technical development. Most importantly, it was largely Australian. Trainor also knew and respected John Gough, who was CEO of Pacific Dunlop until 1987. Gough shared many of Trainor's philosophies, believing that decision-making should be delegated to the groups, subsidiary companies and various factories. It was vital to keep outstanding people in the company to develop them and encourage them. It did not matter whether they had been to university. 'Good people come from anywhere,' he would say, reflecting Trainor's own management philosophy.

Thus in 1988, when Nucleus held more world patents than were held in every field by the CSIRO and with 1700 people working for him, Trainor was grieving and ready to sell. In a letter sent worldwide to Nucleus and Telectronics Holdings staff on 25 July 1988, he wrote:

> My dear fellow colleagues and friends, with the support of my fellow Directors and close working colleagues, we have been able to choose a suitable partner to take us into the 1990s and beyond.
>
> Our proposed merger is with Pacific Dunlop Limited, an Australian Public Company with Shareholders' Funds of $730 million, Sales of $2623 million and Net Profit of $140 million at 30 June 1987. They have a long and successful history and attached is a summary of Pacific Dunlop.
>
> We had identified in 1987 in planning for growth of the Company to significantly increase our equity base and our financial strength,

such that we could grow to a One Billion Dollar company by the 1990s.

The Trainor family (representing 50% of Nucleus) had insufficient funds to carry the growth effectively into the future, and dilution of the Trainor family equity would leave the Nucleus Group and hence, Telectronics and Cordis Pacing Systems, vulnerable to hostile takeover. This must be avoided.

So, we sought a partner who, strategically, would have the following characteristics:

- *Had a proven track record of growth in revenue and earnings*
- *Understood and could relate to the international markets and offshore manufacturing*
- *Was financially strong*
- *Held the same high ethics as our Group to the clients, staff and shareholders*
- *Would give autonomy to our Executives in the Nucleus manner*
- *Would compensate and reward staff fairly*
- *Would preferably be an Australian Public Company, and hence relate to the origin of the Nucleus culture.*

We studied a large number of companies and institutions and selected Pacific Dunlop. We advised them of our strategy and invited them to make a fair offer to the shareholders to acquire the shares in Nucleus, which also controls 53% of Telectronics Holdings Limited.

Pacific Dunlop's reaction was positive towards such a merger, and indeed, favoured the theme of also acquiring the balance of shares in Telectronics Holdings Limited at a fair price to the shareholders.

Pacific Dunlop has independently watched the progress of the Nucleus Group over the past seven years and could assess the benefit of a merged fit due to:

- *International marketing and manufacture*
- *The window of the extremely high technology competence*
- *The similarity in management style and ethics*
- *The opportunity to enter the growth field of the Scientific Health Care industry.*

Strategically, it is the right fit.

The Directors of Nucleus Limited, and separately, Telectronics Holdings Limited, independently reviewed the terms of the 'offer' to ensure that the best interests of the shareholders were considered. As the Interim Results were due, the Directors decided to accelerate the release of the Interim Results to ensure that all shareholders were fully informed.

A joint News Release by Pacific Dunlop, Nucleus and Telectronics is attached. The formal documentation starting with a Part A Statement by Pacific Dunlop will commence this week and if all goes according to plan, a Formal Offer will be made in August.

I, on behalf of the Trainor family, fully endorse the recommendations of the Directors and genuinely believe it is in the best interests of the shareholders and indeed in the best interests of all personnel.

At a time mutually agreed, I shall fully retire. However, I personally will be available at any time to provide counsel and support to the Directors and Executives of Pacific Dunlop and to Dr Jim Loughman who will be the CEO of Nucleus. I have highly recommended Jim to Pacific Dunlop and Jim has graciously accepted this heavy responsibility. This provides continuity in management and culture and all who know Jim, know that he cares for the Company and the people and is responsible in looking after shareholders' funds.

There is definitely no plan to change structure nor roles in the Nucleus Group, other than Dr Jim Loughman holding both positions of CEO of Nucleus and Telectronics Holdings.

I have a healthy respect for the policies and performance of the Directors of Pacific Dunlop and for their key Executives.

On a personal note, there is no ulterior motive – I am A1 in health (well A2 at my age of 61) ... I shall continue to work for the Australian Government in various roles and be accessible to Jim (but not interfere). I wish to spend some quality time for myself and with my family.

So, subject to meeting all the regulatory requirements and the acceptance of shareholders, this should all be in place by late 1988.

In the meantime, let's not 'yak yak' but let's 'do do do' to achieve our budgets for 1988. You have done well in the first six months – let's excel in the last six months to 31 December 1988.

My sincere thanks to all the loyal shareholders and staff who have been with me over the bad times and the good times. A new era is to commence and I am pleased that I will be able to witness it. (Think of the bloody alternative!!).

Signed: Paul M. Trainor

Trainor gave away much of the wealth he gained from the sale. Of his $60 million, 20% established a trust for medical research, 20% was distributed to select staff (some of whom had been with him for two decades), 10% went to charity and 10% was given to friends. He decided to set up trustees to manage and distribute the wealth, following his philosophy that it was not good for the kids to have too much to themselves. 'It takes away your work ethic', he said 'and it doesn't do much to develop your life, leaving you exposed and in danger.' His two sons appeared to agree that it would be imprudent to be left with more money than anyone could handle.

With his sons' blessing, Trainor decided to donate about $12 million to others. He had never run the company as a 'boss'. 'I kind of run it more motivationally', he said, 'but then taking the helm and leading. And I act as a wisdom pit to give some guidance when it is needed.' Thus many of the staff were not really surprised at the distributions – having known him for many years, they understood that that was the way he was. 'I don't think many of my senior colleagues, indeed many of the colleagues I work with around the world', Trainor said, 'would be avaricious. The kind of people I work with are in it for health care.' From his perspective, their loyalty needed to be rewarded.

The merger of Nucleus and Telectronics with Pacific Dunlop was completed in 1988. It was a large takeover involving $190 million in cash and shares. Paul Trainor, the controlling shareholder of Nucleus and the controlling Chairman of Nucleus and Telectronics since taking equity, having created Domedica, Ausonics, Cochlear, BGS (Bone Growth Simulator) and Medtel Pty Ltd, sold the lot to Pacific Dunlop and retired completely from the business.

CHAPTER 11

A global conglomerate rose and fell: Pacific Dunlop

Sir Leslie Froggatt wrote his last entry for the Pacific Dunlop annual report in 1990. He had served on the Pacific Dunlop board for 12 years, a period that saw enormous growth for the company. Throughout that period, from 1978 to 1990, the company survived the 1970s' turmoil of simultaneous high inflation and high unemployment as OPEC and the microchip enforced paradigm shifts in economies throughout the world. By the mid 1980s fortunes had turned and economic opportunities for global companies such as Pacific Dunlop expanded as the Australian dollar was floated and the Australian labour market steadily began the shift to deregulation. By 1987 Australia had enjoyed four to five years of very buoyant conditions and relatively high domestic growth. Housing starts were at record levels, commercial property construction was peaking, tax cuts had increased disposable income and the climate was generally one of optimism and expansion.

In these heady economic conditions, the directors of Pacific Dunlop announced the purchase of Nucleus on 25 July 1988. They reported that the company had acquired, on a cash and shares basis, an approximate 18.34% interest in Nucleus Ltd, a world leader in scientific health care technology and products, and that it would make offers on a cash and shares basis for all remaining ordinary shares in Nucleus and its 53% owned subsidiary, Telectronics Holdings. In respect of both offers, a fully successful acquisition would require the issue of approximately 32.6 million Pacific Dunlop shares (of which 4.5 million were issued in July in respect of the 18.34% interest already acquired) and cash payments totalling $28 million. The offer for Nucleus was declared unconditional on 19 September 1988, with Pacific Dunlop then being entitled to 60.6% of Nucleus' issued capital.

At the time, Pacific Dunlop had probably the widest collection of popular brand names ever held by one Australian company. Its consumer products included Slazenger, Grosby, Holeproof, Bonds, Birds Eye, Edgell, Peters, Four'n Twenty Pies and 15 other well-known brand names. Its automotive sector owned brands such as Goodyear, Beaurepaires, Dunlop, Marshall Batteries and eight others. Building and construction divisions included Sleepmaker, Dunlopillo, Tontine Industries and nine others. In distribution it owned Repco, Checkpoint and another six brands. Pacific Dunlop had 69 brands in total; it was a significant conglomerate that had grown by progressive takeovers over many years. Initially involved in the making of tyres, throughout the 1980s Pacific Dunlop had extended into a myriad of interests and takeovers of established firms. It was not fazed about purchasing Nucleus for $190 million.

The management and directors of Pacific Dunlop had considered two questions in their decision whether to buy the Nucleus Group. First, was Nucleus worth buying? Second, did Pacific Dunlop have the managerial and technical skills to make the most of its purchase? The first question was easy to answer. The Pacific Dunlop board considered that Nucleus was a bargain, hopelessly undervalued by the share market. Even at $190 million in cash and shares, Nucleus was still a bargain by world standards. Of course, the board knew there were risks. The line of business was quite new to Pacific Dunlop and therefore outside its guidelines for expansion. Here, the brand names were not important. The acquisition of Nucleus would not easily fit into the company's internal circuit of transfers whereby talented administrators moved to a new product and soon felt at home. However, the purchase was a clear opportunity to move into a new area with positive future growth, well within the company's stated objective of acquiring businesses that operated in the global market and were the best in their industry.

Paul Trainor had been confident in his choice of acquiring company for several reasons. Pacific Dunlop had the cash to sustain Nucleus' growth. It was Australian, but had an international focus and the skills to ensure growth, thereby ensuring the health of the medical devices industry in Australia. It operated under a structure of divisional management with a philosophy similar to his own. Furthermore, he was confident that the senior management team at Nucleus had more than enough capacity to run the company when he was not around. His successor, Jim Loughman, was an amazing man to whom Trainor was very close. Loughman had drive, he had a low handicap in golf, he played a saxophone, he had charisma and he was very capable. Trainor was also confident in his two top line executives, Robert Foot who headed Operations and Bill Thomas who headed Finance. Backing them were the seven top executives who ran each of the companies which formed the Nucleus Group. Trainor had expected that Loughman would run the operation with a drive and a philosophical underpinning that matched his own. He also expected that Loughman would run Nucleus independently, answering to Philip Brass, CEO of Pacific Dunlop.

Not all Trainor's assumptions matched the expectations of Pacific Dunlop. The management of Pacific Dunlop in 1987 had the cash and was experienced in international commerce, but the company's overriding philosophy was increasing shareholder investment. That meant protecting shareholders' interests at all times and not being afraid to dispose of non-performing assets. Economic rationalism rather than nationalistic entrepreneurship was the driver. It didn't take long before this critical difference affected the Nucleus group of companies.

The first challenge to the newly acquired group came in the changing economic conditions. By 1989, only months after the transfer of ownership, the economic downturn became quite severe. In Australia this meant some painful government policies, including very high interest rates. When Froggatt retired from the board there was no indication of how long the recession might last, thus global companies such as Pacific Dunlop faced a particularly demanding management task if they were to maintain growth for shareholders.

Froggatt wrote that although the annual figures showed positive evidence that Pacific Dunlop would survive the difficult times, the previous year had been a sobering experience as the company refocused and reduced some of its operations. Maximum emphasis had been placed on productivity improvement in consolidating the gains of recent years.

The annual report of 1989 said, 'Your board knows that conditions will still be difficult in many areas but after last year we are an even leaner, more competitive company. We believe the company's policy of making the most of offshore opportunities and focusing on international competitiveness within our business remains vital for the future.' The economic jargon and focus did not augur well for Nucleus. Its non-core companies were threatened with liquidation even though in 1989, its first year as part of Pacific Dunlop, Nucleus had contributed profit of $22 million before interest and tax on sales of $210 million. One of the first subsidiaries to receive notice was Ausonics. Pacific Dunlop consultants considered that it wasn't a core subsidiary and therefore should be liquidated. The Head of Operations, Foot, was able to convince Brass to give him time to develop the company until it was ready for sale. Five years later the sale was made and another Australian company left Australian shores, this time to Israel. Foot left the Nucleus group with the sale of Ausonics. Other Nucleus companies, Domedica and the Bone Growth Simulator (BGS) soon followed in Ausonics' footsteps.

Philip Brass, CEO of Pacific Dunlop, fully supported that economic assessment of the situation. Brass had been appointed Managing Director on 11 December 1987, succeeding John Gough who resigned to take up the appointment of Deputy Chairman of the board as part of a succession plan to replace Sir Leslie Froggatt on his retirement. Brass was originally a shoe man. Brought up in Melbourne by his grandparents, he worked on Saturday mornings at his uncle's shoe stall in the street markets. He enjoyed the challenge of selling and demonstrated very early a remarkable capacity for handling financial details. He completed a Commerce degree at the University of Melbourne, working during his holidays for Hollandia Shoes. Hollandia was bought by Pacific Dunlop in 1968 and Brass stayed with the new firm, rising quickly to General Manager of Grosby Footwear at the age of 26. Brass was in his early 30s when, as manager of all Pacific Dunlop's footwear, clothing and textiles activities, he became a member of the main board. His policy in clothes was to move the company out of high fashion, out of men's suits, jackets, manchester and almost everything that was expensive and instead manufacture clothes with brand names, low prices and big sales volumes. A strategy of high volume, low price and brand names was almost the complete opposite to the Nucleus approach to a manufacturing structure.

Another blow to Trainor's assumptions about the operation of Nucleus within Pacific Dunlop was the death of his successor, Loughman. Within a few months of the sale, Loughman, always a heavy smoker, was diagnosed with lung cancer with brain secondaries. He resigned almost immediately from all participation with the company and was replaced by Thomas, a finance man brought into Nucleus from Sharp in the early 1980s. Brass found Thomas to be very able, handling finances with expertise and very much to Brass' satisfaction. This was a critical change for Nucleus. The company was now seen through economic rather than medical engineering eyes, and that would badly affect both Telectronics and Pacific Dunlop in the next four years.

Brass was increasingly impressed by the Nucleus staff's enthusiasms, knowledge and desire to make the best possible product. But he confessed to colleagues that he saw them as scientific dreamers. They were utterly absorbed in the technology of their products. They did not want profit for profit's sake; they wanted profits only to survive. He did concede, however, that their skill in inventing, in manufacturing and in selling had earned them remarkable success. But Brass' view demonstrated the unfortunate change in focus for the medical group.

By 1990, as the recession began to really bite, the Pacific Dunlop strategy of consolidation took on a major role and ideas of expansion receded into the background. The consumer business became particularly difficult in Australia, where the economic downturn was quite severe. As a consequence, the enhancement of shareholder value took on a new emphasis. Company priorities became working capital control and extracting cash from under-performing assets. Capital needs were curbed, inventories and accounts receivables were brought under tight management control and gearing was pulled back to 46.5%.

The company's consolidation strategy operated through close monitoring of monthly financial reports relating to sales, profits, inventories, profit margins, cash flow and projected earnings. There was no room for concern about the widely varying cultures of the very diverse divisions, as long as their earnings, cash flow and inventories remained satisfactory. It was a very turbulent period for Nucleus people. In their business, it made no sense to get inventory down. That is a suitable strategy for a high-volume, low-margin business where it is possible to build up inventory very quickly, but in the production of highly technical items a lost sale of one unit in Telectronics or Cochlear would mean a loss of $5000–$10 000 of margin. It makes little sense to keep inventory low, when the costs of keeping inventory are not nearly as high as the costs of losing supply of the product.

In addition, during this time of cost-cutting Pacific Dunlop regarded R&D as discretionary. In its experience, capital expenditure meant building factories: that was its understanding of building capability. There was little understanding that R&D was the high-tech equivalent of capital expenditure in an environment where it was critical to have high R&D expenditure. That was the company's capability. Constant pressure to reduce R&D and cut back expenditure on it produced disconnections on how to run the medical devices business. Such disconnection was unfortunate: the whole reason for selling Nucleus to Pacific Dunlop was to gain the funding that would enable Telectronics to continue innovating products. As Nucleus' expansionary needs collided with Pacific Dunlop's consolidation policy, the disconnection in strategy led to some serious problems.

Possibly the most serious and ultimately disastrous dysfunction appeared in 1990. In that year Brass insisted that the medical group, then led by Thomas, place its product development and marketing on a more commercial footing. R&D programs were shelved if they fell outside the core business areas of pacemakers and hearing implants, and the focus turned to market rather than technology drivers. The problem was in the USA where Nucleus had difficulty bedding down its $33 million acquisition of the pacemaker division of Cordis Corporation. Cordis had developed a bad image because of product recalls of implanted devices, and its name was dropped in favour of the Telectronics brand. Finally, the axe had to fall on one of the company's two pacemaker manufacturing sites, with Miami winning out over the sentimental favourite Sydney, to lower costs and improve access to major markets in the northern hemisphere. The move was also intended to increase specialisation – a good strategy for the manufacture of low-cost consumer goods but not necessarily the best strategy for the manufacture of high-value medical devices. The move required the transfer of processes which had been based in Sydney for 25 years. The head office of Telectronics was moved from Sydney to Denver.

Brass had the long-standing view of Australia as an attractive place to perform R&D, early production and market development, especially for a high value-added product, but believed that 'When a product is mature – and pacemaker technology and the pacemaker market was now growing only slowly – logic dictated a move to the US.'

Brass and Thomas shared the view that international players in any technology type of industry eventually had to establish their base close to their market. In 1991, their considered opinion was that Australia would be a lot better off from what had occurred. Brass stated that after about a year local manufacturing would return to its present level as younger products gained wider markets, and that profits would flow in from the USA.

Unfortunately, the benefits of knowledge transfer from working in technology clusters, developed by Trainor over 25 years, were completely discarded. Manufacturing moved from an organisation with a careful culture and no product recalls in 30 years, to one that had developed a bad name through recalls within the industry. When the networks were merged, close to 200 people simply left the Australian company – a devastating loss to the Australian high-tech industry. Trainor refused to comment publicly on the move but it must have broken his heart. A contemporary observer noted the change in Nucleus culture. On the boardroom wall at the Nucleus medical group, small display cases proudly showed every model heart pacemaker made by the company since 1963. Every model, that is, until the 1988 takeover. Under Pacific Dunlop ownership, Nucleus lost the paternalistic touch of Trainor. No one bothered to put the company's latest pacemakers in glass cases. The 200 jobs lost in Sydney only underlined the sad changes in the company perspective.

The economic rationalistic approach also discarded the benefits of Trainor's technological nursery concept. Trainor was proud of nurturing up to 100 R&D projects at any one time. Some, like the bionic ear hearing implant, were spectacularly successful. Others were failures, such as the scientific computer abandoned after $1 million was spent on development. Trainor insisted that there should always be products in development and the approach must be very long-term. He constantly emphasised that it took 10 years to develop the bionic ear. It took 25 years to develop the original pacemaker. It was very hard work, but there always had to be nursery products in the system. Trainor highlighted Cochlear in Nucleus as an example. It was a project under the Nucleus umbrella, then was incorporated as a subsidiary. It lost money and lost money, but in the context of a plan. It wasn't just burning cash and hoping for the best. The opinion formers had a plan that involved developing the product to get the clinical outcomes although for quite a few years the rate of expenditure was much greater than the rate of revenue. That was the advantage of a nursery concept – being under the Nucleus umbrella gave Cochlear and other companies under development a foundation because Nucleus had profitable companies such as Telectronics and Domedica to provide support until the project could become a successful stand-alone company. The strategy was, however, an expensive one.

Moving Telectronics to the USA in 1991 initially appeared to be a success. A substantial growth in sales and profit validated the potential that Pacific Dunlop had seen when it acquired Nucleus in 1988. The newer rate-responsive and dual-chamber pacemakers at the high end of the market were launched and Telectronics recovered its share to 10–12% of the world market. US FDA approval was received for a Meta single-chamber-rate responsive pacemaker; 1300 were implanted worldwide by the end of the year. The Meta dual-chamber rate-responsive pacemaker began clinical trials in the USA and the FDA approved the Reflex single-chamber pacemaker for commercial sale. The advanced Guardian 4210 pacing defibrillator began clinical trials in the USA. To 1991, 600 defibrillators had been implanted worldwide. The Pacific Dunlop 1991 annual report stated that 'the economic trough has become deeper and more protracted than many people expected. Sales in most businesses other than the Medical division were either static or lower and development of the Medical division's manufacturing and product development priorities had put it on what appeared to be a strong growth path for the future.' The medical division was expected to be ready to contribute significantly to profit, but those expectations were short-lived. That was the last positive report card for Telectronics.

As Ausonics struggled to realise its saleable potential and Telectronics struggled with restructure, Cochlear also had trouble adjusting to the new regime although it continued to grow with increasing returns, albeit less quickly than Pacific Dunlop expected. Cochlear was a smaller component of Nucleus, but under Trainor's leadership it had expanded throughout the USA and Europe with increasing sales generating a growing revenue stream. It was already the international market leader for cochlear implants and it had good scientists and able technical managers in Sydney. So Mike

Hirshorn was excited to receive a phone call from Thomas early in 1989 telling him that David Money, CEO of Cochlear, was receiving a promotion and that Thomas would like Hirshorn to take on the role of CEO. Hirshorn had just returned from the USA and Europe, where he had developed a good reputation in marketing. He had hired the team in the USA and Europe and knew that they would work fantastically together, especially if there was more emphasis on marketing than engineering.

Thomas urged Cochlear to grow at a faster rate. With Money still on the Nucleus team, the plan was to get the benefit of Money's experience and allow Cochlear to benefit from faster growth through Hirshorn's marketing experience. Financially, 1989 was a very good year. Sales grew from $14 million at the beginning of the year to $22 million at the end of the year. A new speech processor had been launched before Hirshorn became CEO: every release of a new speech processor means growth for several years because implantees usually like to buy the newer model. His sales figures benefited from that technical advantage.

Although the year was very good for Cochlear, Thomas was not happy with the monthly financial reports. This was a new culture for the Cochlear team. They had always operated with tight budgets but the emphasis was on changing lives not cutting inventories and minimising costs. It was a highly stressful situation for Hirshorn. Monthly reports in Pacific Dunlop required much more reporting than had been needed before. Hirshorn pondered the question on what lobbying Cochlear had done to increase the level of protection for Australian manufacturing. This was totally foreign to Cochlear, which was about global penetration rather than tariff barriers. Pacific Dunlop was clearly a very different business with very different expectations. Hirshorn didn't do the reports very well. He left them to his CFO, who was also having trouble adjusting to the new regime. They were always behind and there were mistakes which reflected on Hirshorn. Relations between him and the CFO declined, and the CFO departed. Hirshorn employed a young South African, Neville Mitchell, who had very sound commercial experience, but it was perhaps too late. Despite the growth and the profits in Cochlear, there were complaints from direct reports and a lot of frustration with Hirshorn's performance in that area.

At the end of the year Hirshorn was informed that there would be a reversal of the changes made the previous year; Money would be reinstated as CEO of Cochlear.

It was proposed that as Hirshorn had been such a success in setting up Cochlear in Europe and the USA, he should take on Japan as a challenge and develop the south-east Asian market. The news that he was to lose the position of CEO was a real blow to the ambitious Hirshorn, but he took the new challenge and successfully opened up Cochlear in Japan.

The 1992 annual report announced a disappointing performance for the medical group, claiming that it had been affected by unexpected operational problems. Those who had lamented the Telectronics restructure were not surprised. Medical group earnings for that year were lower because of difficulties with a small number of new model pacemakers. Although Telectronics had established itself as one of the world's most reliable manufacturers of implantable pacemakers and leads over the previous 30 years, during 1992 it had difficulty with a small number of newer model pacemakers. These problems were rectified, but they incurred considerable costs in notification, warranty and change. Telectronics tried to keep operations going and successfully released the Meta DDDR dual-chamber rate-responsive pacemaker. It received FDA approval for commercial release in February and thus had a full contemporary range of pacemakers to market. The next annual report noted that 1993 was largely a transitional year for the medical group as it concentrated on product development in its three core businesses.

Cochlear showed excellent growth results for the next four years. Cochlear hearing devices had a record year in 1993 and the company continued its very significant expansion in all geographical locations, with unit sales of 1678 making a total of over 5000 units implanted worldwide. The expansion of the children's implant program in the USA in particular was rapid, exceeding adult implants for the first time. Successful implants in patients with severe hearing difficulty, as distinct from those with a profound hearing disability, created another market that was recording pleasing results.

The next year, 1994, was also a good year for Cochlear. For the first time, Cochlear not Telectronics headed the annual report with record sales. Money retired to his preferred position in R&D and Catherine Livingstone, previously CFO for Nucleus, was appointed CEO. During that year Cochlear devices received Ministry of Health and Welfare reimbursement approval in Japan, which was expected to add significantly to future sales. The new Spectra 22 speech processor was successfully launched worldwide and yielded excellent results. By 1995 Cochlear was the shining star in the Nucleus group, achieving an excellent result with sales increasing by 24% and profits by 18% annually. Cumulative implants of Cochlear systems exceeded 11 000. Adding to the list of successes for the period, the company received approval from the FDA panel for cochlear implants for the severely hearing impaired. The clinical trials of next-generation Micro implant and companion speech processors, including a behind-the ear-speech processor, also provided continuing opportunities for growth. However, despite Cochlear's stellar performance since 1988, Pacific Dunlop reported in late 1995 that it planned to divest the company.

The rationale for the decision was Telectronics' devastating performance, brought on by two crucial events – FDA questions about manufacturing processes and the failure of a small lead in its pacemaker. By 1995, the Nucleus group as a whole was suffering badly. Board member David Penington noted that within two years of him joining the Pacific Dunlop board, the Telectronics team was in dispute with the US FDA over aspects of its manufacturing following a routine inspection. A combative and legalistic stance in dealing with the FDA could refuse the company permission to manufacture or sell its products in the USA. Despite Penington urging Telectronics to work with, rather than against, the FDA, the company's stance changed little. Its earnings were still very good at $354 million and confidence was high, so Telectronics was very confident of its position. It continued to assume that the problem with the FDA was based on hostility to the fast-growing Australian share of the US pacemaker market and ignored the consequences of taking a confrontational stance with a regulator, especially one as powerful as the FDA. Penington knew of another pacemaker company, which had worked its way out of serious jeopardy by close consultation with FDA at every stage. Telectronics management was unwilling to follow that approach. Its combative approach unfortunately led to Telectronics having to enter into a Consent Decree with the US FDA on compliance issues related to FDA concerns about the maintenance of good manufacturing processes in the USA. Manufacture for the US market was suspended while the necessary corrective measures were undertaken.

Before the difficulties with the FDA were resolved, the company was hit by real disaster. A small number of injuries and two reported deaths occurred in patients implanted with its pacemakers. A small wire named the Accufix 'J' lead, that held the electrode tip against the muscular lining of the atrium of the heart, had suffered metal fatigue and fractured. This design feature had been acquired from Cordis. Outrage in the media was followed by a US class action against Pacific Dunlop based largely on 'fear of failure'. Fewer than 10 fatalities were finally identified, compared with more than 40 000 devices implanted and functioning well worldwide, mostly in people with serious heart disease. However, the FDA had no reason to assist Pacific Dunlop given its combative approach and, as the class action gathered momentum, Telectronics was finished.

The class action was a crippling blow to Pacific Dunlop. The large multi-national was already under serious pressure in terms of falling earnings in its diverse divisions and a falling share price. Despite heavy expenditure in the new food division, it was losing money. The battery division in Columbus, Georgia, a huge investment in an imaginative but complex battery recycling plant, was in trouble. Heavy expenditure in tyre manufacturing in Melbourne failed to turn this around. Price reductions imposed by motor manufacturers were a problem for both. Public sentiment was turning against conglomerates. Pacific Dunlop made the decision to sell its recently acquired food division, at a loss, and the class action over pacemakers was the *coup de grace*. Within several years Pacific Dunlop, under a new chairman, was shedding most of its subsidiaries and its proud title disappeared.

The unfortunate consequence of Pacific Dunlop's fall from grace was the destruction of the Nucleus group of companies. Ausonics had been sold, Domedica, the Bone Growth Simulator and Medtel Pty Ltd were disbanded or sold and although the liabilities of Telectronics was an ongoing problem for Pacific Dunlop, it was no longer a proud Australian pacemaker company. Only Cochlear survived the turmoil. It prepared for sale, with a new leader at the helm.

CHAPTER 12

An Asian expansion became necessary: Japan

In 1994, shortly after Catherine Livingstone took the reins of Cochlear within Pacific Dunlop, Cochlear proudly announced that it had managed to obtain Japanese Ministry of Health and Welfare approval for reimbursement of the Cochlear hearing device. This was excellent news and no minor achievement. When David Money returned to the role of Cochlear CEO in 1990, replacing Mike Hirshorn, Hirshorn's new job was to get Japanese approval for sale of the implant in Japan. A survey of medical device companies demonstrated that Japan was an enormous and very lucrative market. It was anticipated that Cochlear would achieve good results and a major effort was made to ensure that this occurred.

Initially there had been correspondence between Professor Graeme Clark and Professor Sotaro Funasaka of Tokyo Medical University, who had been very impressed with Clark's presentation at a conference in Melbourne. Funasaka eventually observed surgery in Melbourne and did some practice on temporal bones with Clark and his colleagues. The first bionic ear operation in Japan was performed on 7 December 1985, by Funasaka, on a 41-year-old adult. This was a major milestone in a country that was traditionally cautious about implanting devices into the body. Funasaka was a major champion of the Australian cochlear implant in Japan. He trained and inspired other doctors, including Professor Kohzoh Kumakawa, who was a younger doctor at another hospital.

However, taking the cochlear implant business to a commercial level involved many questions about how to start. Important questions included the most appropriate distribution method, methods of training people and prospective office locations. It was a formidable task, but Hirshorn enjoyed such challenges and he had a record of succeeding at them. He visited Japan for a week every month, for two years. A whiteboard was installed in the company's tiny office and on it was written 'Ready', 'Set' and 'Go'. 'Ready' was for when they had completed all the required documentation. 'Set' was getting an import licence and 'Go' was for when they received the reimbursement. In 1994 Cochlear was ready and set to go.

There were really only three ways of trading in Japan at the time. One was to appoint a distributor who had an import licence. The second was for a company to have its own subsidiary and get its own licence, and the third was to appoint a Japanese caretaker company. The Telectronics experience had shown that if a Japanese company was appointed as a distributor, it could be very hard to transfer its import licence back to the company if a change was required. If the company chose an inappropriate distributor and wanted the licence transferred, for instance, the distributor was under no obligation to do so and would not want to lose face, thus the company might get stuck with the wrong distributor. It could be very destructive. Such an event had happened to Telectronics and Hirshorn didn't want it to happen to Cochlear. The caretaker option would have been useful: a genuine caretaker company would take responsibility in Japan for all Japanese activities. It would be paid, but there would be no payment for the set-up and all the costs incurred in the many years it takes to get an import licence. It took Cochlear seven years to gain an import licence. That's a lot of costs before any revenue is generated. However, although the caretaker option was publicised in the law and regulations advice for the industry, investigation showed that it had never been used. In the late 1980s it only had the appearance of being an alternative path. Today that path has been used and there are caretaker companies in Japan, but it was not an option for Cochlear at the time. The only choice open to Cochlear, therefore, was to have its own subsidiary and get its own import licence.

Fortuitously, the opportunity presented itself through Telectronics, which had been operating in Japan for some time as Nihon Telectronics. When Telectronics acquired Cordis in Florida, distribution for pacemakers in Japan changed from Nihon Telectronics to the Cordis distributors. This change in direction presented an opportunity to acquire an import licence through a subsidiary. Hirshorn was able to easily convince Money of the benefits and the Nihon Telectronics staff helped to manoeuvre Cochlear through the regulatory environment to buy the company which became known as Nihon Cochlear. But getting the licence for Nihon Cochlear involved Ministry of Health and Welfare (MHW) approval, which meant very detailed documentation of clinical trials on the safety and benefits of the implant. The documentation from the US FDA approval process was in English and could be translated, but there were literally thousands of pages. Also the Japanese MHW was not willing to just accept foreign data. It wanted local data, including results from Japanese clinical trials, but was reluctant to specify the number of patients for whom data were required.

There was a further serious obstacle to carrying out clinical trials. It was impossible to import the necessary equipment without an import licence, and it was impossible to get an import licence without clinical trials on patients. Funasaka had been able to carry out cochlear implants by successfully applying for a grant to purchase and do the first implants, but someone still had to get them through customs. The hospital could not assist. It had no mechanisms for importing devices for doctors.

Dana Japan was a distributor of audiology equipment in Japan and an importer of hearing aids. Hirshorn asked Funasaka who he thought would be a good importer of the Nucleus cochlear implant. Funasaka said, 'Well, Dana Japan supplies me with all this other equipment and we have also co-developed a product for auditory brain response equipment. We have worked closely with Dana Japan, so I think that they might be a very good importer even though they are a very small company.' He introduced the Cochlear team to Dana Japan and its Director and Chairman, Shuzo Kimura. Dana Japan provided the assistance necessary to clear the devices through customs and delivered them without difficulty since Funasaka was already a customer. It was a very valuable relationship, all done on a handshake. There was an agreement that when Nihon Cochlear had its import licence it would compensate Dana Japan for the work; for many years all the work was done without payment. Like Trainor, Kimura was an entrepreneur. He owned the company and could decide to supply the implant in the hope of getting paid in the future. It helped to build relations with a customer, and there weren't many implant patients. There were only 30 devices imported over several years, which was manageable, but Dana Japan's assistance was critical to the survival of Cochlear in Japan. Cochlear had consulted other distributors of medical equipment and visited bigger companies, because Dana Japan was only small. The bigger companies were interested but Cochlear decided that they might not give its product as much attention. Also, they were mostly importers. Dana Japan, on the other hand, was a manufacturer of audiology equipment. Cochlear decided that the smaller company would be technically much stronger and therefore able to service the surgeons better. It was a very good decision.

Hiring a CEO for the new subsidiary was also a critical task, but one with which Hirshorn had a lot of experience. He had employed all the subsidiary CEOs so far. The person he appointed for Nihon Cochlear, Hajime Noguchi, was the right person for the important task of achieving the licence and reimbursement objectives. Noguchi, a former employee of Johnson and Johnson Japan, had the correct demeanor and attitude to help gain MHW approval for the Nucleus Cochlear implant. Hirshorn and Noguchi worked with Shinichi Watanabe, the new subsidiary's chief technical officer, who had done a respectable job as acting CEO until Noguchi was recruited. Watanabe had worked with Nucleus in Nihon Telectronics, ensuring it retained its import licence, and kept in touch with the MHW. He had translated documents of clinical trials into Japanese for Nihon Telectronics but the number of documents from the Cochlear FDA approval process was huge. He started to do the submission to the MHW but could not develop a good relationship. 'They were not kind,' he told Hirshorn. Translating all the documents would cost so much money it was impossible. Nihon Cochlear argued its case with the MHW and ended up translating only the important portions.

There was some awareness of cochlear implants in Japan and 3M already had patients. Not everyone believed the device would work, but at least they knew it existed. The awareness meant that some doctors were already interested in the concept and were willing to be trained to do the operation. The MHW insisted that the trials begin but continued to procrastinate on specifying the number of successful implants that would satisfy the safety requirements for a licence. Negotiations led to the decision that nine patients were required, but when the data were submitted the MHW did not accept that number. It said that more were required. The MHW wasn't sure what number would be safe and politically it was easier to say no than yes. The Nihon Cochlear team found it very frustrating. Funasaka became very angry and helped the lobbying effort. The MHW eventually agreed to accept data on 30 patients, which was manageable since Nihon Cochlear had already implanted 25 patients.

The results were good and, together with the translated FDA trials on 85 patients, they provided substantial evidence of safety and benefits. The product quality was very good and there was a lot of satisfaction for patients and doctors. Nihon Cochlear was a very happy team and very relieved to finally have the implant accepted by the MHW, because until that step was achieved it wouldn't be able to sell products in Japan. But the story wasn't finished with an import licence. There was still the question of health insurance reimbursement.

The implant's price in Japan was much higher than the US or Australian price to allow for the anticipated reduction that would come with the Japanese import licence and reimbursement. The rationale for the price centred on the Japanese method of health insurance reimbursement, which was complex. At the time, doctors who prescribed drugs also sold the drugs. It was in the doctors' interest to charge the highest possible price and the government would repay them through reimbursements. Doctors made a lot of money from prescribing drugs. The government would deduct a certain percentage from the price every year, and it was expected that the same would apply to the Cochlear implant. The team at Nihon Cochlear knew that they were entering an environment in which, no matter what price was charged, the government would work on reducing it. The cost of marketing in Japan was higher and operation and office costs, when there is very little revenue stream, were also very high. Therefore the initial price in Japan was set at three times the US price. Although it was very costly for patients, the team knew that the government would reduce the price via reimbursement. They didn't know how much the reduction would be, however, and had to ensure that it would still be economical.

To get reimbursement, it was necessary to negotiate with every hospital to take up the program. Funasaka's recommendations helped with this. Once an operation was completed, the government would pay the hospital, the company would invoice the hospital and then it would be straightforward. But first the MHW had to agree for the reimbursement to begin.

After four years of lobbying, Nihon Cochlear was invited to meet the MHW to discuss reimbursement. It was asked to bring all the documentation on the trials, the devices, the duties paid to customs and all the transfer prices between Cochlear in Australia and Nihon Cochlear in Japan. It was also required to supply the invoices from Cochlear to the hospitals. The meeting was held not in the MHW building as expected but in another building, which was empty. This was very unusual. Everyone met on a floor which was bare except for half a dozen chairs in one corner. It was a strange situation, but MHW representatives went through all the documents and made notes. From this inspection they determined the price which would be reimbursed and, as expected, it was a reduction on the company's original price. It was clear that the strategy of charging a higher price was correct. Did Nihon Cochlear get reimbursement approval at an unofficial secret meeting? It was hard to tell. There were many events that led to the reimbursement approval, any one of which could have tipped the scales in the company's favour.

There were many influences. Building relationships in Japan was critical. Nihon Cochlear constructed a chart listing all the influences, the most significant of which were the data, the documentation and the translations of other countries' clinical trials. But there was always the need to consider all the incidental factors critical for the success of Ready, Set and Go.

The ENT academy in Japan had been asked if it would recommend to the MHW that approval for reimbursement should be given. One day, a letter from the head of the academy arrived at Cochlear in Australia, and its contents generated much discussion. The writer said that he was a collector of butterflies and that his collection included some butterflies from Papua New Guinea (PNG). He had bought them from a distributor from PNG and thought that the butterflies were not of good quality. He wondered if the reason was that the people in PNG remembered the Japanese in their country during World War II. Maybe he was getting inferior butterflies because he was Japanese? He asked if Cochlear in Australia could purchase and send him butterflies that were of good quality, and listed the Latin names of everything he wanted. 'Is this a form of bribery?' they wondered in Sydney. 'Is it just a favour? What should we do? If we get him the butterflies, does this mean reimbursement? If we don't get him the butterflies, does this mean no reimbursement?' They decided to get the butterflies somehow. However, quarantine regulations prevented the importation of PNG butterflies into Australia. The idea of bringing them into Australia then sending them to Japan wouldn't work, so they contacted the Australian consul in PNG and said, 'Look, we know this is not helping PNG–Australia relations but if you can help us you can help Australian exports to Japan,' and explained the request. The consul agreed to see what he could do. Cochlear bought the butterflies but, as only one company had export permission for butterflies, it had to buy them from the same company that supplied the professor in the first place. The butterflies were sent to the Japanese professor, who wrote back that the quality of the butterflies sold to the Australians was no better. But Cochlear still got the reimbursement. Who knows the impact of such events on the decision to approve reimbursement?

The team at Nihon Cochlear drew on many relationships. Hearing a US speaker at a Japanese conference talk about doing business in Japan and his experience in lobbying for US pacemakers, it became obvious that Cochlear would need someone from the Australian government to lobby the Japanese government. There was no one in Australia really who could do very much. The USA had three people lobbying the Japanese government on behalf of US medical devices companies. Eventually, Hirshorn met with Ed Rozinski, who was in charge of the Health Industry and Manufacturing Association in Washington, an industry representative body for health manufacturers.

'If we have a subsidiary in the US and the American subsidiary joins the Health Industry and Manufacturing Association, can you represent us in Japan?' Hirshorn asked. 'No, that's impossible. We are dealing at the top level of the MHW to lobby for the American industry.' The Association eventually realised, however, that the Nihon Cochlear implant was only a very small market, that lobbying could improve the cochlear implant market in total and that it wouldn't cost the Japanese government much but would allow it to say it was approving foreign devices in Japan. Roziniski agreed to use Nihon Cochlear as a case study to lobby MHW. He introduced the Cochlear team to the top level of the MHW, much higher than the level they had managed to reach themselves. Prior to his lobbying, the MHW didn't want to talk to Cochlear at any high level.

AUSTRADE also helped. The head of AUSTRADE, Greg Dodds, had been a trade commissioner in the past. He introduced Nihon Cochlear to a number of people, including a Minister in the Japanese government who was interested in Australia. This was a man called Yasuo Fukuda, who eventually became Japanese Prime Minister. Fukuda's influence could also have been helpful.

An additional source of influence was a Japanese princess, Nori-no-miya Sayako (now Sayako Kuroda), whose visit to Australia in November 1992, including Cochlear's Australian office, gave Cochlear the credibility in Japan to inadvertently help the import licence and sales effort. She was the daughter of the emperor and was interested in people with disabilities. She was well educated and quite controversial, being independently minded. On her trip to Australia she visited only three places – the Sydney Opera House, the Sydney Japanese school and Cochlear. Nihon Cochlear still has pictures in the lobby of her with Hirshorn, Jim Patrick and the Japanese consulate in Sydney. Her endorsement was invaluable. It showed Japanese doctors that the Japanese princess was interested in Cochlear in Australia, so it must be all right. The precise influence of such an event is unclear, but it must have contributed to the acceptance of the company in Japan.

As in the USA and Europe, Nihon Cochlear found that Pacific Dunlop head office in Sydney sometimes didn't understand the obstacles to growth from a Japanese perspective. Livingstone, under pressure from Pacific Dunlop, would insist on knowing why Nihon Cochlear sales were so small. The team tried to explain that Japanese doctors do not change easily, that they have to be convinced step by step. Negotiations in Japan took many steps. They took time. Livingstone wanted the team to push harder, but in the Japanese culture that would not be good. The pressure to increase sales was intense and the targets were very high. Big education programs were organised to help the situation and every day patient or doctor groups in each area were addressed. It was a very busy and very stressful time, but all the bills continued to be paid. Noguchi and Watanabe were never tempted to leave – the challenges were big and the patients were many and it was very rewarding. Watanabe in particular was determined to do the job. He was totally motivated by the patients and their transformation after receiving an implant.

CHAPTER 13

A saving grace emerged: Catherine Livingstone

Leo Port looked Catherine Livingstone in the eye and said, 'Catherine, your mind is like a spreadsheet with a thousand rows and a thousand columns and you know every number in every square and if they don't add up in the bottom right-hand corner, you can't sleep at night.' 'You're right', she replied. The Cochlear team had gathered for a weekend management workshop, where people were paired together for an exercise that involved looking directly into the eyes of their partner and telling them something about themselves. Port had drawn the CEO and had to tell her what he thought of her – on this occasion, she agreed with him.

Livingstone came from a banking family. She had qualifications in finance and was a registered chartered accountant. She had decided that she wanted to get wider experience in industry before returning to the profession and ultimately to academia. She had heard about Nucleus from friends and secured a position there in 1983, working for Bill Thomas and Paul Trainor in a corporate accounting role. She learnt a great deal from Thomas. Livingstone said, 'We had words very often and we had lots of difficult moments on a professional basis about how something should be handled', but Thomas taught her well.

When she joined Nucleus, Cochlear was only one of a number of projects under the Nucleus umbrella. One of her jobs was to find the cash from Nucleus to keep the project going. Nucleus was burning cash on R&D at an alarming rate on the various projects that Trainor kept taking on. David Money, CEO of Cochlear at the time, often visited Livingstone in her Nucleus office, saying Cochlear needed more money. She would reply that there wasn't any. Despite the drawbacks, they managed to keep the project alive.

Livingstone didn't feel at a disadvantage although she was one of the very few women in the company. Like everyone else, she had to prove herself to Trainor. Having demonstrated her financial skills to Thomas, he offered her a promotion. She happily accepted it, and planned to take a month's leave before starting the new job. Just before she left for her break, Thomas apologetically told her, 'Actually, there is going to be an advertisement in tomorrow's paper for your new position.' The very position that Livingstone had just accepted. Thomas said that Trainor considered her to be insufficiently experienced for the role. Thomas had a different view, but Trainor was the boss. The position was advertised.

Applications arrived and the selection process began. Livingstone, frustrated, watched the applicants as they passed her desk on their way into an interview for her job. It could have been humiliating, but eventually Thomas told Livingstone, 'Actually, we will give you the job after all.' That was good, but the salary offered was lower than the one that had been advertised. This was another strategy of Trainor's to keep people on their toes. He would quite often dangle a bait then take it away, believing that if he made life a little bit more difficult for people then a culture of complacency would not develop. Despite this 'character-building' exercise, Livingstone stayed on at the lower salary. Like many others who worked with Trainor, she didn't leave. Her father had taught that 'There's no room for moods – just deal with your problems.' She lived by that advice and went on to great things, eventually leading Cochlear to stock market success.

Thomas and Livingstone worked as a team for 12 years. Together, they overcame many financial hurdles for Nucleus and had many successful outcomes. They worked with the government to receive an R&D concession. Through Nucleus, they championed an R&D syndication. Although the mechanism was subsequently abused by other organisations, if left intact it would have been very useful for businesses such as theirs. They also contributed to the development of the Managed Investments Scheme and the Management Investment Program, from which Cochlear ultimately benefited. The debt was paid back to the government just prior to listing on the stock market. Their achievements required extraordinary efforts but gave them some terrific highs and the impetus to keep achieving.

After the sale of Nucleus and Thomas' promotion to CEO of the Nucleus Group, Livingstone was promoted to CFO of Nucleus. By early 1994 Pacific Dunlop was no longer enchanted with its move into the medical devices market. The outcome of moving Telectronics from its technically sophisticated and effective Sydney operations to the US market for economic reasons, was proving to be a disaster. The Pacific Dunlop board decided that it no longer wanted anything to do with medical technology, but by then only Telectronics and Cochlear were left of the Nucleus Group. Telectronics was a problem that Pacific Dunlop was trying to manage. Cochlear wasn't a problem – it was in fact generating revenue and recording increasing returns on an annual basis – but, having been given a clear indication of the possibilities of future problems in such an industry, the Pacific Dunlop board decided to get rid of it anyway. There would be either a trade sale or an initial public offering (IPO).

In the midst of this turmoil Livingstone became CEO of Cochlear in 1994, replacing Money, who was finally able to return to his preferred technical role. It had taken Money a year to convince Thomas that an exciting engineering challenge existed for the company and that he, Money, could serve the company better in leading the research than by continuing as CEO. Thomas finally agreed to the change, and they discussed possible replacements. Livingstone was their first choice and they offered her the position. She was expecting her third child and said, 'Let me get through the pregnancy and if everything is all right then yes, certainly.'

In June 1994 Livingstone commenced her new role with a brief to get the organisation ready for an IPO in three to four years. Immediately, however, problems with the Cordis 'J' lead really started to escalate. Telectronics also had other problems with its defibrillator and some of the dual-chamber pacemakers. Major problems were erupting, and by November 1994 Pacific Dunlop had had enough. It wanted to get rid of Cochlear by the end of the year.

The CEO's brief changed dramatically between June and November. The new brief added difficulty in requiring Livingstone to simultaneously ready the company for both an IPO and a trade sale. Pacific Dunlop asked whether Livingstone could manage it. 'Well, if someone asks me if I am up to it', she responded, 'there is no way I am going to back down.' The challenge was interesting but the question was unwelcome.

She immediately set the company on a path that would achieve the parallel objectives. The next year, 1995, was extraordinarily stressful as Livingstone had to gain in-depth knowledge of all elements of the business. Her parents had always emphasised the importance of professionalism, reiterating that, 'If it's worth doing, do it properly'. Cochlear in 1995 was a small company with a turnover of less than $100 million. There were no layers of management to which she could delegate, so Livingstone had to understand the financials, the manufacturing, foreign exchange, markets in an ever-increasing number of countries, and the technology. Having an excellent memory helped, but it was a very complex business. Despite this, Livingstone knew where she was taking the company and she was determined to get it there.

The financial control was tight because it had to be. There was no option but to get the balance right. The company had to have money to invest in essential R&D for the new product systems, for marketing and for continuing global expansion. Cochlear was expanding into new countries all the time, and it took a lot of valuable resources to get through the regulatory approval process and clinical trials which were different for every country. It was critical to get the finances right. The company had always operated under tight financial conditions and Money had handed Livingstone a financially viable business. However, prior to 1995, although the company had strong financial discipline it still operated with a research focus. The company officers did the books, knew the numbers and conducted strategic planning meetings, but always in the context of a division of a division of a division. Livingstone was the one who introduced the commercial accountability that was required once the company was exposed to public scrutiny. Public reporting made a big difference to the processes and level of information required. In addition, as the business expanded the manufacturing supply chain had to be streamlined to cope with the increased demand.

Adding to her problems, Cochlear's two main competitors – Advanced Bionics and Med-El – released two new multi-channel systems. Cochlear's market share dropped almost overnight although an 85% share was maintained. Not only was the new CEO trying to guide the company to an IPO in a very short time-frame but the company began to face increasing competition. This had to be rectified if the company's planned IPO were to be successful. Livingstone tried to keep the company on track while working with Pacific Dunlop and multiple advisers and lawyers. She did not share her problems with her team. She shared them with David Penington, the incoming chairman, and Neville Mitchell, who was Cochlear's CFO. She was determined to spare the other senior executives the stress so that they could concentrate on growing the business, which was critical to stabilising trends and retaining Cochlear's position.

The senior management team under Livingstone included Mike Hirshorn, Ron West, Monika Lehnhardt, Neville Mitchell and Jim Patrick. Hearing that Cochlear was going to be sold, some of the management team who had grown the company from 1983 thought there might be an opportunity for a management buyout. Hirshorn became increasingly excited at the thought that if Pacific Dunlop didn't want to own Cochlear anymore, perhaps the management team could provide another option. Emboldened by the prospect of ownership of a company that had driven their existence for over a decade, Hirshorn set about making an appointment with Philip Brass, managing director of Pacific Dunlop.

Hirshorn rang Brass, whom he had known as a child. Brass appeared to be receptive to Hirshorn's idea and told him to come to Melbourne to discuss the proposal. Brass himself set up the meeting and, although he couldn't be there, he sent a representative. Full of anticipation, Hirshorn flew to Melbourne and even bought a new suit for the occasion. He met a small group of Pacific Dunlop senior managers and put the view that a management buyout of Cochlear would benefit the company. He then returned to Sydney. However, Pacific Dunlop was not receptive to Hirshorn's proposal. It was losing millions of dollars from Telectronics court cases and was not interested in considering any option other than the sale of what was left of the Nucleus Group.

Livingstone had difficulty working with Hirshorn. She was CEO, and naturally expected respect for and loyalty to that position. Hirshorn was not the CEO but he behaved as if he was. The pressure of events meant that Livingstone, as CEO, needed to lead the agenda. Team members, if they were going to work for her, had to respect that they were not the CEO and give loyalty to the position. If they were not able to do so, the only solution was to part ways. After a final disagreement which tipped the scales, he was escorted to his office to gather his belongings and, as was the fashion of the day, was shown off the premises.

In a hastily convened management meeting to announce Hirshorn's departure, there was silence as Livingstone outlined the circumstances. Janusz Kuzma, standing in the corner, noticed a tear slowly making its way down Patrick's cheek. It was the end of an era. The concept of the tiger team was no more. Like the inexorable flow of a tide, the organisation moved on but Hirshorn, who for most of his adult life till that point had been striving for the growth of the company, was no longer part of its progress.

During the due diligence process leading up to the planned IPO, Cochlear received from the US FDA a heart-stopping warning letter regarding its manufacturing process. It could have derailed the whole IPO process as there was no way the company could go public with that warning hanging over it. Potential shareholders might fear a repeat of the Telectronics troubles, even though this was on a very different scale. The Telectronics problems involved people dying. The new Cochlear manufacturing issue concerned only a batch of 13 devices with incorrectly inserted capacitors. The capacitor would degrade over time and eventually prevent power from reaching the chip. The whole implant would then have to be taken out and replaced with a new one. Although the batch consisted of only 13 devices, the FDA had to make sure the mistake was confined to that small number. Putting together the documentation for the FDA audit was a huge effort, especially considering all the other issues on the table. Cochlear had to assemble all the appropriate paperwork that would prove it was a limited incident and did not constitute any safety concerns. With the company's imminent launch of its IPO, an FDA concern rang alarm bells everywhere and had to be dealt with immediately.

The assembly of documentation was hindered by the fact that Cochlear was such a small company. Everything was paper-based and processes were less robust than they would have been in a larger company. But the FDA had set a time limit and there would be no second chance. Livingstone therefore felt that she had to be deeply involved in organising for the inspection although it was not her core competency. John Parker, a brilliant mechanical engineer who had joined Cochlear in 1994, was in the critical role of Head of R&D at that time. He immediately set about putting rigour into the processes that had been identified by the FDA. Being an outstanding engineer, he understood the issues from a research and design perspective. They worked relentlessly for six weeks and satisfied all the FDA concerns. Under Livingstone's guidance, the whole team kept its cool and corrected perceived defects. There was an almost audible sigh of relief throughout the company when FDA lifted its warning well before the IPO was ready to be launched.

The planned IPO went ahead and the company was floated at $2.50 per share, based on historic earnings, with all PDL shareholders able to subscribe. The price was based on a growth profile of 11–13% but with no real track record. Turnover was small and no one really knew about Cochlear, it was a brand new industry. Having become acquainted with every detail of the company and being highly intelligent, Livingstone was able to speak with credibility about future prospects. Prospective shareholders could see that there was substance to the company, that it would not be a fly-by-night spin-off. Consequently, the share price remained steady in the months that followed the float. With the IPO completed, the board and the management team faced all the scrutiny that affects a public company. On the positive side, no one in the company could blame someone else for lack of funding. There was no Nucleus, head office or Pacific Dunlop to blame for not being allowed to grow the business. The company was on its own. The management team had to regroup and understand that it now had the freedom to make its own decisions, but that it also had the responsibility of benefiting the shareholders.

An additional challenge for the newly listed company was that it had no cash. Pacific Dunlop had taken every dollar. The lack of cash reserves meant that the company had to pay its own way from day one. It hit the ground running because there was no fall-back position. Pacific Dunlop did, however, offer one saving grace. Although it took the cash, it also left Cochlear with no debt. Since the company had been generating revenue for a few years it had an income from its first day. By not having to chew cash on debt repayments and with the additional assistance of some bank loans, there was cash to carry on operations. Within a very short time it was possible to pay dividends because of the positive cash position. It very quickly became obvious that cash wasn't the biggest issue. The real problem was how to grow the company.

One of Livingstone's defining moments was about to arrive. She said, 'I think we can grow much more quickly than this. The 11–13% growth profile that we have listed at is what we have been comfortable with but I think that we can take growth to 15–18% and then 18–20%, in those sort of ranges.' A former head of McKinsey Consultants was employed to attend meetings and facilitate the discussions. Various strategies were investigated and discussions focused on creating a strategic plan that would allow the company to achieve the higher growth profile. More money would have to be spent to achieve the expected outcomes, but Livingstone was convinced it could be done.

The major focus for growth was on improving sales in various regions and on what needed to be done to get those sales. In the 1980s and 1990s the quantities of implants being produced were so small that even minimal automation was unjustified. Only jigs and fixtures were used to help with the assembly. One of the biggest manufacturing challenges was the need to mount a lot of electronic components onto circuit boards for the speech processor. Cochlear had the largest integrated circuit in Australia at the time, and it was a very difficult thing to achieve. If the company were to meet its objective of continued growth, it would be necessary to use faster manufacturing methods. Manual assembly could not meet the increasing level of demand.

The changes therefore included a redistribution of leadership roles. Patrick moved from R&D to Research and Applications. John Parker became Executive Director and Chief Technology Officer. He took over the manufacture of implants and speech processors and was able to grow the department from a cottage industry to commercial production. Leo Port, a member of the original tiger team who had led manufacturing from day one, saw this restructure as an opportunity for himself. Cochlear had never had an IT department and, as manufacturing was now in Parker's hands, Livingstone agreed that Port could head a new IT area within the company. He was delighted, and spent several years growing this integral part of the business.

One inspiration was the development of a speech processor that sat behind the ear instead of in the recipient's pocket or belt with cables going to the ear.

Ernst von Wallenberg and Peter Seligman had discussed the possibility after the company's launch of an earlier model, the Spectra, in 1993. Although the idea had not been embraced enthusiastically in 1993, placement behind the ear was much better aesthetically. However, some sectors of the company were concerned about performance. Performance was paramount, they insisted. 'We don't want just aesthetics. You can get much more battery life and performance from a processor when it sits in your pocket than you can from a behind-the-ear model'. Lehnhardt, on the other hand, said, 'In Europe aesthetics is important and it will expand the market.' She knew that Europeans prioritise elegance and was confident that a behind-the-ear model would sell well there. Livingstone supported Lehnhardt and the decision was made that behind-the-ear placement was the strategy to take. Great efforts were made to ensure that the new processor did not compromise technological performance. The strategy succeeded and the expanding market had a huge impact on company performance, resulting in growth of 18%. After a couple of years of growth at 18% the company decided to demonstrate its ability at a different level, and aimed for 20%. To ensure continued growth, Livingstone was meticulous to the point of obsession about getting every detail correct and making sure that the financial reporting was completely on target. She often surprised many of those who reported to her, with her detailed knowledge of every aspect of the business.

As the company was committed to the life-long maintenance of patients' implants, the device and sound-processing systems were the subject of continuous R&D. A Cooperative Research Centre, linking Graeme Clark's research group in Melbourne, contributed much to the research. The chairman, David Penington, very much appreciated Livingstone's detailed reports of operations. She met all international travel commitments and handled negotiations involving many international phone calls late at night. Penington had no hesitation in granting her leave for nine weeks to take up an Eisenhower Foundation fellowship to explore management in innovative high-technology companies in the USA. This study period led to fresh thinking about the development of Cochlear, which involved the opportunity to buy a division of Philips Industries based in Antwerp, Belgium.

In 1996 Philips had bought Antwerp Bionic Systems, a small Belgian cochlear implant company that manufactured the Laura cochlear implant. Some time later, advertisements started to appear in the ENT News, advertising Philips Hearing Implants as a new company entering the cochlear implant market. It could have been a big threat to Cochlear's position. Philips was a huge company with very deep pockets and was already making medical devices and hearing aids. It had its own chip design and fabrication facilities. The acquisition of Antwerp Bionic Systems was the last ingredient it needed to enter the market very quickly and in a very big way. Philips also had the advantage of worldwide marketing infrastructure in the hearing aid field. Cochlear could have expected the imminent launch of a leapfrog product.

The Philips Industries acquisition was basically an opportunistic purchase. It wasn't about sales – Philips had only made about 200 units and those involved a liability as the device had a design fault which would eventually lead to failure. The strategy was to establish a base in Europe and the R&D group of Philips Hearing Implants eventually became the Cochlear Technology Centre in Belgium. The group was headed by an outstanding engineer, Jan Jansen. He was key to the company's growth strategy in Europe. This excellent group of people would allow Cochlear to acquire a R&D facility in Europe, in the heart of the European market. Cochlear would then have a key presence in Europe to initiate collaborations with key clinics. The Philips group also had some valuable digital signal processing technology that could expand the company's potential.

Following many discussions, due consideration and substantial due diligence it was decided that it made good sense to buy the Philips division. But the acquisition was not easy. There were very difficult and protracted negotiations, night after night for months, between Cochlear and an international company supported by an aggressive team of lawyers and other experts. On one occasion Livingstone and Mitchell walked out of a meeting and went to the airport to fly home; they received a call to come back because the point was being conceded. Then the next point had to be negotiated. The deal was finally done to Cochlear's satisfaction and Jansen eventually came to Sydney to head the Design and Development department.

Having completed the Belgian deal, taken the organisation through IPO, done all the organisational development and got the financial discipline in place, Livingstone decided it was time to hand the running of the company to a new person for the next phase of growth. 'You always need that fresh pair of eyes and you need the new input of emotional energy', she told the board. Like Money, she had effectively taken the company to a point and felt that it was time to hand it over to someone else. A succession of leadership which fits a particular growth period is critical for healthy company progress. In 2000, through the chairman, Livingstone handed the board her resignation and a new growth phase began under another new leader.

CHAPTER 14

Lives were changed: Li Cunxin and his daughter

A red balloon burst and lives were changed. It was a radiant day in Brisbane before the balloon burst. Li Cunxin, immortalised with the title 'Mao's Last Dancer', was visiting the home of his Australian partner in life and on stage, Mary McKendry. In the north-eastern capital of Queensland, in the land Down Under, the weather was clear and warm. There was a magnificent blue sky that had none of the smog experienced in more industrial cities. Li and McKendry had completed a successful tour of Australia's east coast with the Australian Ballet Company and were on the last leg of their journey before returning to the Houston Ballet Company in the USA. Their 18-month-old daughter Sophie and both their parents were there for the last performances.

Li was gently holding the hand of his young daughter as they slowly returned to the rented apartment where a family party had been organised for that night. Along the way, music and the sound of laughing children caught their attention – a bunch of floating balloons tied with ribbons to a gatepost announced that there was a birthday party in the house. Sophie pointed excitedly to the balloons and Li asked the friendly neighbour if his daughter could have one. The neighbour greeted the request with a warm smile, cut one of the ribbons and happily handed the excited child a big red balloon. It was a tender moment as the father gently tied the ribbon to his small daughter's wrist and they continued their slow journey home. In the next 10 minutes, the direction of their lives would be forever changed.

The world-famous dancer had experienced a difficult life. At the age of seven he was taken from his home in rural China, away from his parents and six brothers, to be trained as a ballet dancer with the Beijing Ballet Company. Discipline was harsh and demanding but at least there was food and the prospect of a better future than the hardship of an agricultural labourer's life. Li was given the opportunity to travel to the USA and, once there, made the difficult decision to defect. He survived the heart-wrenching difficulty of defecting from China to the USA and the many years of separation from his parents, and had finally received government permission to visit his parents and family in China. During this visit to Australia, Li's mind was peaceful. He had married and divorced a young US dancer in a short space of time and was now married to his soul mate. Their dancing careers intertwined and they inspired each other to greater accomplishments. With the birth of a lovely young daughter, it seemed that Li's life was on a path that could not be better. However, the path suddenly took a sharp turn that would have defeated a less focused and determined couple.

As Sophie toddled up the concrete stairs to the apartment, her red balloon burst. The sound was so loud, so unexpected that it startled everyone – except Sophie. Other children cried but Sophie just looked bemused, as if wondering where the balloon had gone. The loud bang had no effect on her at all. Li clearly understood that normally a child would be frightened because the sound was so loud and sudden. He had previously suspected that his daughter's hearing was not quite right. He had noticed that sometimes when McKendry arrived home after dancing and called out to her daughter, Sophie would take no notice until her mother came quite close. Then Sophie would respond with excitement. Li had observed that if Sophie had her back to her mother, she would keep playing until her attention was attracted by a shadow or movements – only then would she react.

Li had questioned his parents about whether this was normal. They had had seven sons and said not to be silly. McKendry's mother had eight children and she also told Li that he was imagining things. At Sophie's annual check-up, the doctor and Li tested the child by clapping their hands behind her back. On the second clap Sophie turned her head, which implied that there was no problem. The doctor proposed a feasible explanation of a two-language family. Li's parents looked after Sophie and spoke to her constantly in Chinese and the doctor said that she would soon be coming out with phrases in Chinese and English. Furthermore, Sophie was babbling, making sounds such as 'baba' and 'mama'. Deaf children are silent. Li had deferred to the doctors and the parents with all their experience. But this time, after the bursting balloon, Li told his wife that he didn't care what anybody said, as soon as they returned to Houston Sophie would be tested thoroughly.

Li contacted the family doctor and demanded that Sophie be tested. Again they were told not to be silly, that they were just being paranoid, but Li was not to be deterred. Even as they drove Sophie to the hospital for testing, McKendry was sure that they were overreacting. But within a few hours, the mood had changed. Sophie had had an auditory brain response test which showed that she was profoundly deaf. Her parents sat in stunned silence as the doctor informed them that their child heard nothing.

Neither of them knew what to do. Li had thought that perhaps there was something blocking the ear. Perhaps a middle ear infection or something similar caused the problem and it could be rectified with a small operation? But Sophie had nerve damage and there was no simple operation that could fix it. Her only option was hearing aids, and the stunned parents were referred to the Houston hospital for deaf children.

Li went into denial. There had to be a cure. There just couldn't be no cure. His whole life had been spent looking for the positive, regardless of the hopelessness of the occasion. He could not accept a no-solutions outcome. McKendry spoke first, saying that they should go straight to the deaf school, where they asked a lot of questions although they were still in shock. The staff were sympathetic and advised that the best thing was to put hearing aids on Sophie immediately. Li and McKendry had limited knowledge of the hearing-impaired. They weren't aware that the advice they were receiving would hold back their daughter's progress for two valuable years while they struggled to help her hear.

McKendry had suspected that there was something not quite right with Sophie's hearing but had never imagined that the child was profoundly deaf. It was devastating to realise that in one way her child was very different from the one she thought she had. Their lives would need a complete change. McKendry was overwhelmed with the feeling that the family had been living an illusion and immediately understood that there was no time to waste — it was obvious that Sophie had not heard anything for 18 months. At the front of the mother's mind was an overarching determination, 'Sophie has to be able to speak to me. She just has to be able to speak.'

Without delay, Sophie was taken to the hearing school and had hearing aids fitted and within a few months McKendry gave up her dancing career so that she could dedicate herself to Sophie's therapy. She felt that she couldn't live with herself if her daughter had no voice. Her perspective was that the voice is part of the person. People have a personality when they are silent, but it is not the same personality when they speak. A person who cannot speak can communicate with only a limited number of people using sign language, and the mother desperately wanted her child to be part of the whole communicating world. She wanted Sophie to be able to communicate in China, the land of her father. Chinese sign language is not the same as Australian sign language, which is not the same as US sign language, and sign language does not always relate to the written word. McKendry knew that Sophie would need to learn sign language but she was also desperate to hear her daughter's voice.

It was very difficult and quite devastating for McKendry to give up dancing. Ballet was what she loved. She had loved it since she was a little child and she had worked hard to reach the top of the profession. The decision to give it all up prematurely was very painful. The decision also affected Li's dancing, because McKendry had been such a perfect partner. He knew how much she loved ballet and what a sacrifice it was to stop dancing, but it was something that she wanted to do for Sophie. Neither McKendry nor Li dwell on the negative. They are the kind of people who just move on. Their philosophy is that once you make a decision, you live by that decision. Looking back cancels the ability to look forward, so they both kept their focus on the outcome they wanted from this new and overwhelming problem. Therefore, although it was very hard on both of them, McKendry eventually changed roles to become Li's coach and his trusted sounding board.

For two and half years Li danced and McKendry dedicated herself 100% to Sophie. They struggled with frustration, trying to make their daughter hear, but she heard virtually nothing. Although she had hearing aids her ability to understand came from lip-reading. They covered their mouths to make Sophie listen, but she seemed to hear only the 'oo's and very low sounds. She was obviously very smart and they could see the determination in her eyes. The process they were following was very difficult but it was the only way they knew that might give Sophie a chance. At every sound she made they leapt for joy. They encouraged her in any way they could and they never stopped talking to her.

In 1992, multi-channel cochlear implants had only recently (1990) been given FDA approval for infants or young children such as Sophie. Fortunately, Collenda Daniels who practised as a speech therapist in Dallas was a strong advocate for the benefits of auditory training. She ran a deaf school and the family was referred to her. Daniels was the first person who asked if they had ever thought of the cochlear implant developed in Australia. They knew nothing about it, and McKendry immediately made phone calls to Australia for more information. The family approached surgeons in Houston and the Houston deaf school and were always given the same firm answer – there was no surgery for children so young and in any case the implant had not been properly approved by the FDA because the concept was still in the experimental phase. This was not quite true, but in Houston the deaf community and the medical profession were against it. The Americans didn't value the Australian research and wanted to do their own. They were not ready to admit that the Australian implant worked. But McKendry didn't want to wait any longer. Sophie was already four and had heard almost no sounds, and the longer her situation remained the same the harder it would be for her. Li and McKendry did their own research; they found that children had been successfully implanted in Australia and that FDA approval for cochlear implants in children had been granted several years previously.

At the age of four, Sophie was taken to Methodist Hospital to be tested for a cochlear implant but the Houston doctors refused to give it to her. McKendry had done a lot of therapy with Sophie, who had thus learnt to differentiate between two syllables. McKendry was convinced that Sophie didn't know what the sounds were or what they meant, but her ability to differentiate them led the doctors to decide she was not profoundly deaf and that an operation could destroy her ability to hear the two sounds. This was not something that McKendry would accept. Her research had shown that a cochlear implant would give Sophie a chance to hear. If the Houston doctors refused to help, McKendry would take Sophie to Australia or Los Angeles where a doctor was performing the operation. Still the Houston doctors refused.

Her response was short and sharp, 'Okay, I'm off to LA.' After several committee meetings with the doctors, speech therapists and the deaf school, the hospital finally gave in but it did not do so lightly.

The family had to sign forms releasing the hospital from responsibility if something went wrong. The pressure was huge. The surgeons were especially reluctant to do the operation; Li and McKendry had to ask many medical friends to lobby them to agree. The responsibility of signing the forms was horrible. Implant surgery was a difficult operation at the time and meningitis was always a threat. The surgeons would not guarantee that the implant would provide any benefit in hearing but Li and McKendry believed that if Sophie were able to hear any qualitative sound they would be able to help her connect to speech. McKendry was giving Sophie so much attention and love that if they could connect her with sound they could connect her with language understanding. Any level of sound that could be provided via an implant would be better than the silence in which Sophie was then living.

On the day of the operation, Sophie was given a doll. The nurse pointed at the doll's ear then pointed to Sophie's ear, to explain what was about to happen to her. After only a few minutes, Sophie understood. It was heart-wrenching for Li and McKendry to watch Sophie's realisation of what was about to happen. She couldn't understand why she was going to be operated on. Why did she have to have this surgery when her parents didn't? Horror filled her eyes and, screaming in terror, Sophie fainted.

The operation took many hours and the waiting was terrible. Although every worst possibility went through the parents' heads, they tried to focus on the positive and talk about when their daughter would hear sound. Sophie woke soon after the operation, confused by all the toys and the people around her, but quickly went back to sleep. Her parents were relieved that she was fine and that the door to possibilities had been opened. The doctors were less enthusiastic, quietly saying that the operation had been successful but that it was uncertain if Sophie would hear any sound. It was difficult to look at Sophie's tiny head and not shed a tear. Half her head was shaved and she had a massive bandage covering 75 stitches. For the next few days every effort was made to prevent Sophie from looking in a mirror.

When the implant was switched on Sophie at first appeared to hear nothing, but she was obviously feeling overwhelmed and cried a lot. Years later she still remembered the experience as frightening and uncomfortable and one that she didn't want. McKendry was present at the switch-on of the program. It took a while to get the channels and levels adjusted but then Sophie reacted as if a light bulb had been switched on. She could hear. McKendry remembers it as one of the most exciting days of her life. If Sophie could hear sound, McKendry firmly believed she could do the rest with her daughter.

A gifted technician undertook the task of programming or mapping Sophie's hearing. McKendry and the technician watched the blinks of her eyes and how she moved in the chair, to understand the sounds she was hearing. Sophie couldn't tell them anything as, without sound, she had never learnt to speak. She just looked at her mother and responded to the various sounds and they guessed at her reaction. The mapping outcome was amazingly good; it didn't require much change over the years. Within three weeks of the implant being turned on McKendry knew that her daughter would be part of the hearing world.

The excited parents had little idea, however, of the difficult path ahead. Five years later Sophie was tested and found to be well below the speaking age of other children. She had lost four years of language development. Progress had been difficult and often disheartening. Sophie could hear sound, but that was only the start of some truly hard work. Every connection she made between a sound and the language and the meaning of that sound was a major breakthrough. At the beginning, virtually every discovery was painful. McKendry would bang pots and pans behind Sophie's head to help train her with sound, and ask whether Sophie heard it. She and Li continued to cover their lips so that Sophie couldn't lip-read, and Sophie kept pulling their hands away in frustration.

McKendry never gave up her determination to give Sophie the best possible chance to operate in the hearing world. Because of her physical background, McKendry was convinced that there was a physical reaction to hearing and comprehending. She could see the physical reaction when information entered her daughter's brain. If she couldn't see that physical reaction, she would start again.

It took a great deal of patience and physical energy to communicate with Sophie. As far as McKendry was concerned, it was possible to talk and to teach without physical energy but it would mean little to the listener. A hearing person would absorb some meaning but a person with an implant would have to attend; the teaching required energy and had to be interesting to keep their attention. McKendry sang, she spoke with a lilt, and somehow she provided constant therapy. Within 12 months Sophie was babbling like a brook, although no one but her mother could really understand her speech. There were many gaps, basically because Sophie's language development had started so late. Learning to read took longer because Sophie had no connection between the written and spoken word but the family persevered although progress was slow. McKendry never stopped talking and Sophie never stopped learning.

In 1995, after dancing with the Houston Ballet for nearly six years, Li decided to join the Australian Ballet Company as a principal dancer and the family moved to Melbourne. He was 34 and nearing the end of his dancing career, but some of his most satisfying performances were during his three years with the Australian Ballet. Australian audiences just loved Li.

The move to Melbourne was difficult but there were compensations. Australia was McKendry's home land and there were people who knew and understood her and who could provide valuable support. When tests showed that at nine years of age Sophie had a speaking age of 2.9 years, it didn't stop McKendry. Other accomplishments, such as Sophie beginning ballet, continued to give her hope. One of McKendry's childhood friends had a dance school in Melbourne, had great empathy and was confident that she could teach Sophie to dance. Not wanting Sophie to miss out on an activity that many little girls enjoy, McKendry and Li allowed Sophie to be taken under the ballet teacher's wing. She proved to be a perfect teacher for Sophie and understood what McKendry was trying to do. Sophie was placed on the front barre so that she couldn't just follow what the other girls were doing. The teacher clapped out the beat, forcing Sophie to listen. She made Sophie understand that there was no other way if she wanted to operate in the hearing world.

There were many anxious moments. Li remembers a performance where the girls were doing a free movement exercise with three long ribbons – when the music stopped, they also stopped. Sophie sometimes stopped in time with the music, perhaps from memory rather than from hearing, Li thought, but sometimes she continued moving when the music stopped and realised her mistake only when she saw the other girls had stopped. Music is easier than language to respond to because of its rhythm; in language, each sound needs to be heard. The ribbon dance showed that Sophie could not reliably hear even a simple rhythm. This worried her parents. Sophie loved to dance but Li and McKendry knew that the ability to dance well depends on being able to hear the subtleties, the intricacies and the mood changes of music. For a dancer, music is everything. The anxious moments, however, never deterred them from persevering.

As well as being good discipline, ballet allowed Sophie to express herself in a creative form that helped develop confidence, especially as she was good at it. Ballet was in her blood and it did not depend on verbal skills. Music and dance allowed her to be the same as and sometimes better than her peers. By the time Sophie was 12 she had the confidence to lead 30 girls in a tap dance routine. McKendry could see that Sophie's brain was ticking over and was convinced that it was only a matter of getting the information into it. If Sophie could lead a group of girls in a dance routine, McKendry was sure she could do anything. The achievements kept coming. Sophie learnt the cello and then the piano, at which she did well, and McKendry was relieved to see her daughter's life expanding.

The more intelligent a child, the more frustrating is the lack of hearing because they are unable to make connections. Sophie often had dark moods. She was frustrated by her lack of comprehension, especially on social occasions like a birthday party. If there was loud music, Sophie couldn't hear the host telling children to finish a game and go to the next activity. She would continue playing, then realise nobody else was there and she would go into a rage. As a young child, Sophie's personality was very dark. She was unable to communicate verbally how she felt, and her rages were a way of telling those around her that she was frustrated.

At nine, however, the level of Sophie's frustration began to fall and she became more confident. Her decreasing rage episodes may have been partly due to her exhaustion. She was working hard to catch up with her language, get through the school day, go to ballet and other activities – there was no energy left for anger. The effort was paying off, however, and not only was she progressing but she was catching up to her peers on several levels. Her skills increased and she was able to express herself better, but she was often still lonely. Because she didn't have the great gift of language she spent a lot more time with her brother than with playmates.

There are a number of causes of profound deafness. These include accidents that cause hair cell damage in the ear, and infections such as meningitis. A recessive gene in both parents may cause their child to be born profoundly deaf. Li had a cousin who was deaf and, although McKendry was not completely sure, there may also have been deafness in her family in the distant past. Having borne one child with profound deafness, the decision to have a second child was fraught with anxiety. Li and McKendry knew they were taking a huge risk, but agreed that it was the kind of risk that was worthwhile. Although there was a 50% chance that a second child would also be deaf, they believed that Sophie should have a sibling. Without one, Sophie's life would continue to be lonely – something that the parents, both from large families, agreed was too terrible to consider.

Tom was born in 1992. His hearing was tested and proved normal. Sophie loved her baby brother and, later the sister who was born in 1997. She had no resentment of a new baby taking attention away from her. When she spoke of Tom, her eyes lit up. 'He's perfect', she would say. He was her toy, someone to play with. Sophie was three when Tom was born, old enough to nurture him and want his company even at her speech therapy sessions. Consequently, Tom spoke in fluent sentences at 13 months. He and Sophie developed a beautiful relationship. He was Sophie's friend when she had no others, he was her protector, he was never antagonistic and he always understood her. When she said the wrong thing, he would help her by correcting it immediately. Having a second child also reduced some of McKendry's focus on Sophie and eased the tension for them both.

McKendry seldom let Sophie be looked after by anyone else, concerned about the huge responsibility. A babysitter would have to watch Sophie all the time. If Sophie were called, she wouldn't hear. However, there were two people who Li and McKendry trusted to look after Sophie. One was McKendry's friend Annie, who also had a little girl. The Li children spent a lot of time with Annie and her daughter because it was very safe. Another source of comfort was Sophie's godmother, who took the children every Saturday and minded them in her back garden which had a massive pool. Saturday was McKendry's break from talking.

From Year 4, Sophie attended Melbourne Girls Grammar. She had a hunger to learn and the school offered enormous educational support, the staff going out of their way to help Sophie given her hearing limitations. Unfortunately, by Year 7 the changing group dynamics meant that Sophie was suffering socially. McKendry studied the playground situations and realised that 12-year-olds tended to walk, sit and converse in a line abreast. Most of the time, Sophie couldn't hear the conversation and the topics changed so fast that it was very hard to keep up. Sophie would get upset, but there was not much that she could do about it. McKendry noticed that the groups of girls gathered in circles rather than lines as they got older, but the conversations were still too fast for a hearing-impaired person.

It was not only group dynamics that developed Sophie's feelings of isolation. When she started at the school in Year 4, she had not been able to hear or speak very well. That situation changed as her speech improved but despite her increased ability she continued to be pigeon-holed, and was very unhappy. McKendry wondered whether Sophie would like to go to a different school and have a fresh start. Sophie also thought she might do better in a new environment where people wouldn't think of her as she had been in Year 4, but in the end she opted to stay at Melbourne Girls Grammar because the teachers were fantastic. They knew exactly what she needed and how to provide it. They used an FM radio system which allowed them to talk to Sophie via a microphone to cut out background noise, and they knew her moods and how she learnt. Sophie worried that if she started in a new school she would have to start all over again, which could take months or even years. She realised that she couldn't have everything, and was determined to do well at her current school.

At 16 Sophie was offered a scholarship to attend a Houston school for six months. The principal had known the Li family when they were in Houston and had stayed in contact when they moved to Australia. He took a particular interest in Sophie and felt that his students could benefit from knowing Sophie and her story.

McKendry was very anxious about letting her daughter go to the other side of the world on her own. Although Sophie would be staying with close, trusted friends, they had no experience in dealing with an implantee. The long stay would be the first time Sophie was away from her family for more than a night but the experience significantly contributed to her personal growth.

The school went out of its way to accommodate Sophie's needs, arranging class seating in a circle so that Sophie could see everyone and locate sounds easily. If someone were sitting behind or beside Sophie, she often missed the first part of the question while she tried to find where the sound was coming from. The new classroom arrangement made a huge difference in her ability to keep up.

Li visited Sophie while in the USA on a speaking tour and was delighted to find that she was happy and participating in many activities. She was playing hockey for the first time, as the goalie, wearing a helmet to protect her ears and having a wonderful time. Staff told Li that Sophie had exceptional eye–hand coordination, which was perfect for a goalie. The academic staff also gave Sophie individual tuition. One of the teachers said, 'Sophie, I don't believe that someone as intelligent as you are can't get the essence of mathematics. I won't allow you not to understand it.' She would teach Sophie for an hour every morning before normal class time, if Sophie was willing. For six months, the teacher gave Sophie that special time and when she returned to Australia her mathematics ability was excellent. Formerly it had been barely average. Mathematics is a logical process and one missed step can make it hard to understand a concept. Sophie had missed many steps in every lesson and there were many gaps in her understanding, especially in subjects like mathematics. The early morning lessons completely changed her level of ability not only in maths but in many other subjects as well. The most valuable lesson Sophie learnt in Houston was how to be confident. Before Houston, her mother had always been at her side and looked after her every need. When she returned to Australia, Sophie had the confidence to start moving to independence.

An even bigger challenge was her desire to speak Chinese, to connect with her Chinese heritage and her father. Li thought that it would be impossible. Chinese is a very difficult tonal language and Graeme Clark told Li that the cochlear implant had not been designed for tonal language. In spite of considerable and ongoing effort, presentation of tones remains elusive. But Sophie was determined. She wanted to speak Chinese. And she did. She studied Mandarin at Year 12 level and her final exam score was in the top 70–80% of the state. Li's parents were thrilled. They spoke no English, and were excited that their Australian grandchildren could communicate with them. To improve her ability in the language Sophie went to China for five weeks and attended a Chinese school. She stayed with a local Chinese family and coped very well.

At 18 Sophie completed her VCE exams. She was ranked fourth in Victoria for ballet and scored well enough in the rest of her subjects to gain a place in the University of Melbourne Bachelor of Environments course, with the intention of continuing to Architecture. She finds it a very different social experience from her school days. At university she is no longer part of only a small group who all know each other intimately. She constantly meets new and interesting people. Sophie is very self-reliant. She sits in a particular spot that picks up FM signals and liaises with lecturers to make sure they know to have the FM radio on and to speak clearly, neither too quickly nor too loud. If they face away from the students too much she tells them to face the front, particularly if the lecture includes something new. The university has a disability department which is a great help to Sophie. The unit provides a tag in some lectures and tutorials if there is so much information that Sophie can only keep up if someone takes notes for her. She is sometimes given extra time for exams, or a separate exam if the subject is based on videos that lack the subtitles that would allow her to understand the information quickly. Sophie's university experience is one of trial and error. Her advisers are helpful but sometimes she has no clue what they are talking about. Sophie finds different ways of dealing with issues until she finds a way that works. She is progressing well.

McKendry and Li appreciate that life will never be easy for Sophie. They are very proud of their daughter's determination and perseverance. Sophie never saw her deafness as limiting her potential; she was always determined to achieve at the highest possible level. Li and McKendry consider the cochlear implant an amazing gift. They believe that, without her implant, Sophie would not be at university and nor would she have been able to experience the full life which helped create her confident personality.

Their praise for Cochlear Ltd includes words such as 'fantastic' and 'incredible'. The Li family recognise that the success of this Australian company is threefold, comprising the implant technology, the support network and the business acumen. The technology was certainly ground-breaking and the company works very hard on R&D to continually improve the technology even though it already has a significant share of the cochlear implant market. But it is not just about the technology. Li sees a real passion throughout the company to make a difference to people's lives.

The passion is clearly demonstrated at all levels from surgeons, bio-engineers, audiologists and speech therapists to administrators. All these people have keenly embraced the technology and built life-long services for their clients around it. For the Li family, the support network was always as important as the technology. Li is convinced that without it, the technology would not have been as successful.

The third element of the company's success is its business acumen. Many Australian companies have started up, entered the international market then failed spectacularly. Not Cochlear. In its 30-year history Cochlear has demonstrated very clear business entrepreneurship to achieve the praise that implant recipients and their families give. It cannot be overlooked, however, that Cochlear benefited from the past experiences of many of its staff who made their mistakes in Telectronics and Nucleus, learnt from them then joined Cochlear and brought their knowledge with them. It is important to know that people didn't always start learning in Cochlear. Their learning started in Nucleus. Chris Roberts, the current CEO of Cochlear, is one such person.

CHAPTER 15

The future is promising: Chris Roberts

Cutting across the heart of Macquarie Business Park, Waterloo Rd leads to the entrance gates of Macquarie University, where it becomes University Ave. As the road curves gently to the left through the tree-lined main drive, a modern glass and steel building bursts into view. On the top right-hand corner of the building is a 2 m high Cochlear Ltd symbol. It is not a sign that is easily missed.

From the top floor of the impressive new building, Chris Roberts is able to view the surrounding sweep of land and its promise for the future. In preparation for proposed development, the current building has features that allow for growth. On the bottom floor of one wing is a corridor that appears to lead nowhere but that will eventually connect to a building that is yet to be built. To the right is another building under construction by the university. It will be the Australian Hearing Hub. Tenants will include Australian Hearing Services and the National Acoustic Laboratories. The plan is far-reaching and full of promise.

The vision is to build a university hearing precinct of several thousand people co-located on one campus at Macquarie University covering the full range of hearing-related services – hearing aids, implants, clinical services to research to early intervention and a whole range of related services. Roberts states, 'Cochlear is a keen member in that opportunity in this business. The hub will house a range of organisations that are currently spread all around Sydney and they are all related to hearing health. It is a unique concept in the world and we will have it here in Australia, indeed here in Sydney.'

Following Catherine Livingstone's resignation in 2000, the Cochlear board, led by David Penington at its listing, commenced a prolonged search for a successor. It led to the appointment of Jack O'Mahoney, who had a background in the orthopedic device industry. However, in late 2002 O'Mahoney indicated that he was not interested in renewing his contract and it was clear that a further change of CEO would be inevitable. At the age of 72 Penington decided it was vital to step down and allow a new chairman to know the company and lead the search for and induction of the next CEO. He was delighted to recruit Tommie Bergman, an experienced company director and electrical engineer of Swedish origin, as chairman. Subsequently, Chris Roberts was appointed as CEO to lead the company into the 21st century.

Roberts commenced his role as CEO and president of Cochlear Ltd on 1 February 2004. His qualifications for the job were exemplary. Roberts was well-known in the medical devices industry as a founding (non-executive) director of ResMed Inc., a leading medical device company treating sleep-disordered breathing, including obstructive sleep apnoea. In 1992 he joined ResMed full-time and until January 2004 he served as executive vice-president and director.

He has been a member of the National Health and Medical Research Council (NHMRC), Australia's peak health advisory body, and chairman of Research Australia Ltd, a non-profit organisation whose objective is to make health and medical research a higher national priority. He is also a member of the University of New South Wales (UNSW) Faculty of Medicine Advisory Committee.

His educational qualifications are just as impressive. He holds a BEng (Hons) in chemical engineering from the UNSW, an MBA and an Honorary Doctorate from Macquarie University and a PhD from the UNSW. He is a fellow of the Academy of Technological Sciences and Engineering (FTSE) and fellow of the Australian Institute of Company Directors (FAICD). It would be difficult to find anyone better qualified to lead Cochlear, with its proud history, to a promising future. Roberts had 20 years experience with the business issues that surround growing international medical device companies and his strong technology credentials were particularly relevant in this high-tech industry. Cochlear's chairman, Bergman, said that the board was extremely pleased to announce the appointment of Roberts: 'He is uniquely qualified to lead the company at this time of its development.'

Roberts' knowledge of Cochlear, its commercial founder Paul Trainor and the philosophical basis of the company was not new. He admired Trainor for many years before Cochlear was even a project under the Nucleus umbrella, and said that

Trainor saw much more in him than he had ever seen in himself. Prior to ResMed, Roberts worked for the Nucleus group in a wide range of positions including vice president of Telectronics, president of BGS Medical, based in Colorado, and CEO of Domedica. Roberts was one of Trainor's A-graders who responded well to challenges thrown at him, and he now leads the only surviving company from the Nucleus group of companies that Trainor worked so hard to establish. It was said that Trainor's companies thrived as a result of his personal motivation and enthusiasm. Trainor died in January 2006 but he would surely be pleased to see the company in the care of his highly accomplished protégé.

Leading this life-changing company is important to Roberts. Cochlear was something that Trainor started and Roberts feels a great sense of responsibility for its future. His appointment was a relief to people who had worked for the company for many years. Having dedicated hundreds of hours to the company, it was good to know that they would be led not by someone driven to move up the corporate ladder and on to another job but by someone who understood the organisation's philosophy. After seven years under Roberts' leadership, there is a real sense of stewardship throughout the firm.

In organisational terms, Roberts had the qualifications and experience to be the right person in the right place at the right time. David Money had provided strong engineering understanding and tight financial management when the company had to survive by creating the best new product in the cochlear implant market without losing financial viability. The ability to stay in business while breaking new scientific ground is a double-edged requirement for firms in this sector, and one that very few scientific entrepreneurs are able to manage. Money handed over the reins in 1994 to Livingstone at a time that required a redirection of focus to commercial accountability as the company made an initial public offering and listed on the stock exchange. The Money–Livingstone handover was a critical changing of the guard at a time when the company needed a new skill set. Having used her remarkable financial skills to list the company and move it to new levels of financial accountability and growth, Livingstone handed the reins to yet another skill set. O'Mahoney did not stay long, but his successor Roberts has the experience and expertise to take the company to long-term sustainability. The road may be rocky but the future is still promising.

Like any company, Cochlear has weaknesses but one of its major strengths is its staff and management team. The Cochlear human resources department does surveys on employee satisfaction, which show that staff do not particularly focus on financial rewards. The remuneration is naturally appropriate for the outstanding skills of the engineers, technicians, clinicians, financial, legal and many other highly skilled staff involved in the extremely complex business, but the satisfaction rating item that is most outstanding, and that has not changed from that of the PhD students working on the cochlear implant at the University of Melbourne (UOM) 40 years ago, is the satisfaction achieved from making a difference to people's lives. The perspective reflects Trainor's perception many years ago that 'Many of my senior colleagues, indeed many of the colleagues I work with around the world, are not avaricious. The kind of people I work with are in it for the health care and its benefits to the recipients.' The satisfaction that Cochlear gives its employees is reflected in the duration of employment. Most of the original tiger team retain some connection with the firm. Jim Patrick, who started with the project in Melbourne in 1975, is still there and still very enthusiastic about the work and the achievements that will benefit implant recipients. 'We still have many opportunities on the horizon,' he said. 'We have come a huge distance but if it is possible to imagine then we can do it even better.' Money, the first CEO of Cochlear, Peter Seligman and Leo Port have all retired from the business but have input into projects. Mike Hirshorn, until his premature death in 2011, chaired the Cochlear Foundation board.

Although it is recognised that a long-serving staff can lead to a culture of complacency, this is counteracted by the changing technological and geographic horizon. Innovations provide many new challenges and employees who are not driven by profit are motivated by seeing a profoundly deaf businessman negotiate a successful deal via his mobile phone. A clinician still has tears come to her eyes when she watches the businessman succeed – he would not have been able to do that without his implant and she has contributed to the process. 'It is the sort of company that grows and does wonderful new things, which makes being here such a fascinating career' is the view of many interviewees, who have been with the company for over 20 years. The employees' greatest satisfaction comes from the positive impact of their work not only on implant recipients but on recipients' families and networks.

Multiply the benefits of the 160 000 implants since 1978 by family members and networks, and the numbers of people affected are truly huge.

Cochlear has stable management teams and long-serving advisory boards that have provided sound advice backed by a thorough knowledge of corporate history and a strong understanding of the business at all levels. Stability also ensures vigilance over long-term issues in the company's R&D strategies with an important balance between the long-, medium- and short-term issues. Roberts is fortunate that his predecessors laid sound foundations for the company and the 10-year aspirational goals that they had for the company have not changed. The company's mission is still to provide sound to people who would otherwise live in a world of silence; to do so, the business must remain financially viable. However, with several decades of growth the sustainability of the mission can be a challenge.

It can be argued that the company's biggest strength has always been the superiority of its product. The ability to win over 95% of market share in 1988 was due to the product being the best available cochlear implant on the market. Other implants enabled a recipient to hear sound, but the Cochlear 22-channel implant allowed a recipient to recognise speech. No longer was it necessary for families and friends to learn sign language to communicate with a profoundly deaf person. Over 20 years later, the company maintains its position as the world's most reliable manufacturer of cochlear implants that can assist the recipient to understand speech although competitors such as Advanced Bionics and Med-El have slowly nibbled at its market share, bringing Cochlear's dominance of the market down to its current 70%. Since 1989, when Cochlear bought its rival 3M, it has maintained a very strong market lead due to the continuing superiority of its product. Since its tiger team beginnings, Cochlear has produced several generations of cochlear implants, each more reliable than the last.

The latest cochlear implant system, the Cochlear Nucleus 5, included the Nucleus CI500 series implant, which was the thinnest implant on the market. Cochlear, known for its impeccable record of implant reliability, noticed an increasing trend in reported failures of the CI500 series implant. Although only a small number of implants were affected, the organisation decided in September 2011 to voluntarily recall unimplanted devices from that series until it could rectify the issue and reverse the trend. In October 2011, the cause was identified as a manufacturing problem which had led to a loss of hermeticity in a small number of implants. When that happens the implant simply shuts down, without injury to the recipient. Fortunately, Cochlear was able to switch to another implant, the Nucleus CI24RE, which is functionally very similar although mechanically different. In the meantime, it continues to work on the CI500 series manufacturing process and looks forward to regaining regulatory approvals for the series.

The challenge from competitors is not minor. Med-El has Australian headquarters in Perth and its implant is said to be quite good albeit simpler than the Cochlear implant, with only one mode of stimulation. Some elderly patients consider the simplicity to be an advantage, as there is only one control to manipulate. The Cochlear system is slightly more complicated, but the speech recognition is very similar. Med-El also offers a slim implant, similar to the Nucleus CI512.

The other major competitor, Advanced Bionics, left the market for a while because of a product recall but announced its return the day that the Cochlear CI500 implant was recalled. Therefore the market is getting very competitive. A cochlear implant is after all a product, and for some years analysts have predicted that there would be copies. The saving grace is the size of the market. Although each slice of the cake is proportionally smaller, the size of the whole cake is so much bigger that growth can be sustained for a long while yet.

Customer loyalty is key to technological innovation and is one of Cochlear's key strengths. The founding CEO, Money, established the ambitious strategy of promising life-long support to recipients. The strategy extended to buying other hearing implant companies that were going out of business, and taking on their liabilities in an effort to keep the industry viable. The strategy has repaid its costs many times – recipients are indeed life-long customers. Cochlear is firmly committed to making the latest advances available to all recipients, including the very first. From 1982, patients have had access to five upgrades in speech processor technology, and enjoy the hearing improvements without further surgery. This is a significant benefit not always shared by recipients of other manufacturers' cochlear implants. Each recipient of a Cochlear device has an individual service record, which provides good sales indicators for future technological upgrades. To maintain continuity of service, Cochlear has partnered over 3000 clinics in over 100 countries and thus can guarantee support almost anywhere. It is partnered with leading international researchers and hearing professionals to ensure retention of its position at the forefront of hearing science. In 2011, Cochlear had more than 120 research projects under way in over 20 countries. As new products are developed, the sales figures improve.

Roberts said, 'Technological innovation is an important driver of our business, particularly given that we are extending beyond cochlear implants into hybrid systems, giving us a tremendous opportunity in this company to come out with a range of products that will add benefit to a large number of people.' The number of prospective recipients is growing for a number of reasons. Geographic spread, an increasing middle class in developing economies, ageing populations in developed countries, government support and technological advancement are all factors that contribute to market opportunities.

Geographic spread has always been a company objective. Trainor and Money knew that Australia would always be a very small market, which is why Hirshorn was sent to the USA in 1984 with a $10 000 cheque and a deceptively simple instruction to set up centres wherever he thought they could be successful. Another key strength was Money's insistence that nationals understand their own market better than anyone else. Thus an American, Ron West, was chosen as the first US CEO. This philosophy continues. Every Cochlear CEO has to balance the need for regional autonomy with the need to maintain head office directives. It is not a challenge that threatens Roberts. Having been an overseas CEO he understands the challenge and considers that increasing Cochlear's global distribution is one of the company's biggest opportunities. The company has worked hard to diversify geographic sales with emerging economies. These, particularly China and India, now account for a good proportion of all unit sales.

Trainor's effort to establish connections with China have worked well for the company. Chinese government support and a strong private sector model have enabled very respectable growth in the number of implantations being done in China. A bonus appeared in May 2006 in the form of a philanthropic benefactor who promised 15 000 implants to Chinese children. Cochlear thus received an order worth approximately $270 million from a major healthcare organisation based in Taipei, to supply Nucleus cochlear implants in Taiwan and China over the next few years. Korea is also a growing market, particularly since its government started reimbursing for cochlear implantations a few years ago. The number of implantations in India has increased amazingly from a very low base and it is catching up to China. One hospital in India achieved the outstanding result of 18 implantations in one day, which is not only extraordinary in terms of surgery but exceptionally good for extending awareness as well as sales. Implants in India are not funded by the government, however some reimbursement is possible through government agencies and the armed forces which fund not only serving members but also their families – collectively, up to 28 million people. Cochlear expects to benefit from wealth creation in the world's emerging economies with an extra billion people expected to join the middle classes over the next decade. However, projections need to be made with caution. Japan, for instance, appeared to be a promising market in the early 1990s but has proven to be disappointing for a number of reasons. Despite reimbursement and a potentially large market, sales there have been flat for over 10 years.

Opportunities in the developed world involve increasing awareness that will lead to an expansion in demand. Creating awareness of the implant is an ongoing focus for Cochlear. In 1992, the enchanting photo of Pia Jeffery on the back cover of a telephone directory drew the public's attention to Cochlear. The Cochlear implant has been featured on an Australian stamp and the Australian telecommunications company Telstra has produced an advertisement showing cochlear implant children. In the USA, a former Miss America was implanted with the device and promoted its benefits. In each case, positive role models enhanced the opportunities for increasing the company's market. Awareness has been growing steadily and further growth lies in the ability to add value – if someone has an implant in one ear, they may opt for a second implant. Indeed, bilateral implants are becoming more popular for both adults and children. As populations are ageing, the company is only at the very early stages of treating older patients and it expects to expand that market during the next decade.

Cochlear also offers a bone-anchored hearing aid for hearing-impaired people. The device uses the normal hearing mechanism of the cochlea but bypasses the middle and outer ear by vibrating the skull through a titanium pedestal. For many years, the Cochlear Baha System has connected hearing-impaired people to the world of sound. With over 85 000 users worldwide, it is a proven, clinically tested and documented system for treating hearing loss.

The company has also done an enormous amount of work to streamline and improve its supply chain. On the drawing board are ideas that focus on simplifying the process for a recipient. The current practice for repairs is that a recipient must go to a clinic, which then obtains a replacement from Cochlear. The new plan is for the recipient simply to phone and use a warranty replacement process whereby replacements are sent directly from the company. The improved process would save patients' time and increase the treatment efficiency of the health professionals, thus reducing the company's dependence on them. The clinical pathway to intervention has benefited from technological advances and the development of the internet. Cochlear is therefore working on its online and digital strategy, rolling out projects that address remote connectivity to its products and adding transaction tools.

Not all the initiatives to reduce dependence on health professionals have been universally welcomed. Cochlear looked at expanding the role of Australian Hearing into the mapping and programming of recipients, however, the complexities of the financial transactions between medical bodies that this would require prevented the development. Many regions depend on government support in terms of health reimbursements. Strong government support worldwide, particularly for paediatric intervention, is a major factor in people's ability to afford an implant. In Australia the cost of an implant is $25 000, with an additional $10 000 for follow-up services. Such costs can be prohibitive to many people. Where intervention is publicly funded, however, pressures are likely to emerge. Health budgets in developed countries are heavily scrutinised by governments pressured by a myriad of conflicting demands and adverse economic circumstances such as global financial crises. On the positive side, cost–benefit analyses indicate that people's ability to hear and recognise speech allows them to communicate and operate effectively in the hearing world and thus contribute growth to the national marketplace. An inability to hear customers is a formidable limitation to carrying on a business. It follows that such limitations impact negatively on national opportunities for economic progress. Independent studies have estimated that children with profound hearing loss benefit enormously from early intervention, as do governments. Governments save money overall as children with implants can attend regular rather than specialist schools and have lesser reliance on disability services. Sophie Li's story in Chapter 14 demonstrated that assisted children can attend university, which allows them to find better jobs with higher salaries. First Voice, a coalition of hearing-service providers, estimated that every dollar invested in early intervention will return two dollars in social and educational benefits and behavioural improvement.

Such research underpins the need for government support for screening newborn babies in developed countries. Early identification encourages earlier intervention, thus reducing the need for longer-term support. A deaf or hearing-impaired child would grow up in the hearing world and therefore develop language skills similar to those of hearing children. Screening clinics in Australia, however, report that the number of children diagnosed as profoundly deaf is greater than the number being implanted with a cochlear device. When a child is diagnosed, the family is referred to a deaf clinic. The Deaf community remains very cohesive and it may be that the lack of referrals for cochlear implants stems from that part of the process. The strength of the Deaf community's commitment to the status quo was shown on a banner at a deaf school in Christchurch, New Zealand: 'Thank you God for the gift of deafness'. A hearing precinct such as that planned for Macquarie University would help spread awareness and perhaps reduce some negative aspects of the process. However, creating the precinct may not be as simple as Roberts predicts. The SCIC's current site in the grounds of the previous Gladesville Hospital costs the peppercorn rent of $1 per year. At the Australian Hearing Hub it would have to pay commercial rates, which is not an attractive business proposition.

For the Australian government, the cost–benefit analysis is very positive. The Cochlear implant is manufactured in Australia, with exports of the device bringing 95% of the company's revenue with Australia comprising only 3–5% of Cochlear's global market. The bonus to the government of the high export figure is that 90% of the tax that is paid globally is paid to the Australian government at both state and federal level.

Although sustained growth and oscillating exchange rates will always be challenges, Cochlear's low debt and strong cash-flow position with continued investment for the long term augurs well for the company. However, whatever the level of R&D spend, in technology-driven industries there is always the possibility of a new technology that will destroy the demand for current products. Cochlear is not immune to such threats despite its dominant market position. The industry, including Cochlear, is trying to develop a commercially viable and fully implantable device, including battery, processor and microphone, which would have obvious cosmetic appeal. Cochlear has been researching such a device since the early 1990s, with some success.

Early in 1993, Money informed Thomas, then CEO of the Nucleus group, that he wanted to leave his role as CEO of Cochlear so that he could focus on the totally implantable cochlear implant project, which he codenamed TIKI. Livingstone, who succeeded Money as CEO, agreed that TIKI should be the umbrella project for a number of smaller related projects in the company's strategic research program.

Throughout the 1990s, the large external components which were strapped to the body grew smaller and smaller thanks to developments in miniature electronics. Most school-age children and adults with a cochlear implant use a small behind-the-ear (BTE) sound processor about the size of a power hearing aid. Younger children might mishandle BTE sound processors, therefore they often wear the sound processor on their hip in a pack or a small harness, or wear the BTEs pinned to their collar or elsewhere. The possibility of damage is constant. A totally implantable device would avoid the problem. Evaluation of Cochlear's TIKI project has been part of a research project conducted by Cochlear and the UOM under the umbrella of CRC HEAR being the first cochlear implant system capable of functioning with no external components. The system is capable of providing hearing via the TIKI device in stand-alone mode or via an external sound processor.

The project resulted in the successful implantation of three very sophisticated world-first prototypes, beginning on 5 October 2005. Money was on holiday in Western Australia but flew to Melbourne for the first switch-on, leaving his wife and campervan in Kalgoorlie until his return. Many people had been involved in the design and development of the system, but Money was particularly grateful for the two brilliant engineers and enthusiastic champions who drove the project to completion. Helmut Eder in Sydney and Peter Seligman in Melbourne had been vital, both individually and in rallying the large team to success. Not only did the TIKI success confirm Cochlear as the leader in cochlear implant technology, it also enabled the company to evaluate the problems that had to be solved before a commercial system could be released. It is only a matter of time before Cochlear has regulatory approval for a totally implantable cochlear implant hearing system.

Another innovative technology on the horizon is stem cell research, but it could be years before the regulatory system approves the use of stem cell regeneration. Cochlear continues to invest heavily in R&D in order to remain the industry leader and to provide the best results for its growing number of recipients. Trainor was aware of this need, as was Clark. When Pacific Dunlop finally understood what it had to do to stay in the medical devices business, it did not have the vision to make it work. Roberts, following in his predecessors' footsteps, does understand the issues. The company vision – 'Hear now. And always' – appears to be sustainable in the future and demonstrates to the world that it is indeed possible for an Australian medical company to become an international leader.

CHAPTER 16

Software and hardware: development of a clinical system

The history of a medical devices company would not be complete without the story of the product it sells. Between the corporate structure and the clinical outcome lies the product, which requires a lot of engineering. Without product development, there is nothing to sell. The winding and rocky corporate road is matched by an equally winding and rocky R&D road.

A cochlear implant is a piece of implantable electronics but as a prosthesis it is much more than that. A surgical procedure is involved, and much work has been done to refine implantation techniques and reduce operation time from about eight hours to two hours. The length of the incision, the area of hair shaved and the duration of stay in hospital have all been dramatically reduced. In the early days of cochlear implants, children who were implanted still sounded deaf. Outsiders often assumed that it meant the device was not working. Today, many children are implanted at an early age and as a result develop speech of a quality that would have been unheard of a few years earlier. They can now sound like normal hearing children.

The implant system includes an externally worn sound processor, initially called a speech processor. The audiology and programming of the external device are crucial to a successful outcome, and the development of the hardware to perform that task is a story in itself. A considerable engineering effort is required to design and build that hardware, which is manufactured in relatively small numbers since each clinic will have only one or a small number of units. Although the world market for the device is relatively small, the demands on it increase. Each cochlear implant and each sound processor must be compatible to allow clinicians to program not only the implants of new recipients but those of people who were implanted decades ago, again consistent with the company's mantra, 'Hear now. And always'.

The development of software that goes with the programming hardware is also a major project. It must operate with ever-increasing combinations of external and implanted hardware. Over the years there have been developments in sound coding but as not all recipients necessarily can, or want, to use the most recent versions, 'legacy' sound coding schemes have to be supported. This results in a large array of possibilities, all of which have to be under the audiologist's control. The programming options need to be clear, accessible and as simple as possible to use.

The implant can provide feedback on its operation to the audiologist. Electrode characteristics, neural responses and diagnostic information are returned via the software and the results are tabulated and graphed. Software of this complexity requires a team of engineers, and it is an enormous task to meticulously validate each release version and obtain regulatory approval.

The success of a biomedical devices company always depends not only on the quality of its device but on the quality of support and service the company provides. Clinicians have stated that, all other factors being equal, they would use Cochlear on the grounds of the high level of support alone. However, all other factors are not equal. Cochlear is also outstanding for the quality of its implanted hardware, which is several times more reliable than the hardware of any competitor. This is a consequence of its origins in the pacemaker industry and its extremely high level of quality control.

The first Nucleus device was an elegant piece of engineering in its simplicity and it amply fulfilled its role of establishing multi-channel cochlear implants as a clinical intervention. It was, however, only a stepping-stone. With no magnet to hold the external coil in place, the headset was a clinician's nightmare to fit and a constant irritation to the patients. It was also too bulky to be used in children. This first implant was followed relatively quickly by the so-called Mini implant, which had a magnet and was thinner so that it could fit into a shallow cavity in a child's temporal bone. The size was reduced by eliminating the connector between the electrode lead and the implant, to enable replacement of the implant in case of failure. By that time it had been established that the electrode could be surgically reimplanted relatively easily and the connector was deemed unnecessary. The Mini implant was subsequently known as the CI22M and had a production run of 17 000 units, far beyond all expectations.

The Mini was a good implant but researchers didn't stop there. They realised that much stimulation power and hence battery power could be saved by using monopolar stimulation, which allows the inner ear stimulation pulses to flow via an electrode located outside the cochlea. It is much more efficient. More importantly, monopolar stimulation allows the use of much shorter electrical pulses and so facilitates higher stimulation rates. This opened up a world of improved flexibility in speech coding for implant recipients.

To try the idea of an implant with monopolar electrodes, a prototype was made by taking the two highest-pitched, and least-liked, electrodes of a CI22M and using their contacts to connect instead to extra-cochlear electrodes. This simple modification worked well enough to encourage a monopolar trial with a small number of patients but, as sometimes happens, there was a problem. Some of the trial patients received a loud click every time the device was switched on, particularly with the first switch-on of the day. Electronic changes were needed to make it into a clinical product.

Cochlear was simultaneously investigating the use of reverse telemetry. In this, not only is information transmitted to the implant but the implant can transmit information back to the clinician on the state of the electrodes and even whether the neurons are firing. It is a very useful information system for programming children. The new implant was called the Micro, later the CI24M. The '24' referred to the fact that 22 electrodes were used inside the cochlea and two electrodes were employed outside the cochlea.

The development of the Mini implant had been fairly plain sailing. The device worked, and it worked reliably. The company hadn't realised, though, that it had sailed unscathed through a minefield. The Micro development was the opposite – the company ship hit mines everywhere. Patients reported bizarre symptoms and inconsistent results. For example, the first patient reported feeling pain, but only while watching television. Cochlear actually gave him a new television and took his previous one to examine it for possible sources of the problem. Other patients reported constant changes of loudness and the audiologists had great difficulty in measuring the threshold and comfortable levels. In some cases, the start-up clicks were very loud. Thinktanks comprising Cochlear staff and University of Melbourne (UOM) engineers puzzled over what could have gone wrong. Changes were made to the design, but without knowing the specific cause of the symptoms it was always a concern when the new version was tried. Time and time again problems re-emerged. The Melbourne clinic, Cochlear's main trial centre, was losing confidence. Its role was to put patients' interests first and it halted its trial of the Micro. The sales staff were becoming edgy because product development was taking so long; Cochlear was overdue for a new product release and the market was very competitive. Monika Lehnhardt made the decision to find a European clinic that would continue the trial. She found one at the ORL University Hospital in Zürich, under Norbert Dillier, a prominent cochlear implant researcher. Peter Seligman was sent to Zürich to continue troubleshooting with Dillier and his able assistant WaiKong Lai.

Eventually, after a huge effort by many engineers and clinicians, the CI24M was launched as a successful clinical product. A few recipients with the earlier versions of the device are still using it, with special programming attention. The successor to the CI24M, the rugged CI24R, was a mechanical improvement produced without drama. The CI24RE, rugged and with new electronics, also had its moments although they were nothing compared to those of the Micro. The CI24RE, with its improved telemetry and more flexible stimulation modes, was championed by Chris Daly, one of the first Nucleus engineers to be involved with the cochlear implant. It is the current technology and is only the third chip to be used in Cochlear's implants over the company history. It may be surprising, in the rapidly changing world of silicon chip technology, that a new chip is introduced only every 10 years or so. One reason is that the validation and regulatory approval for a new chip is a major undertaking, and very expensive. It is not done unless there is an absolute need for it. Another reason is Cochlear's philosophy of designing implants with a high degree of flexibility. New speech-coding strategies don't usually require new implants and even the earliest implantees can use the most recent sound processor developments.

While the Micro saga was continuing, a new speech processor was being developed, known as the SP5 and later the SPrint. This was Cochlear's first processor based completely on a digital signal processor (DSP). To match the new implant, it used an advanced radio frequency (RF) communication protocol and a higher frequency, 5 MHz instead of 2.5 MHz. To program the new processor, a new computer interface was required. As the new system required new software, four major technical developments had to be achieved simultaneously.

When the Micro hit its first mine, the engineers were in a difficult position. Were patients' bizarre symptoms really due to the new implant? Was the speech processor the culprit? Or the interface? Or perhaps the software? All were new and there was no body of experience to draw on. However, Cochlear, in its thorough and methodical way, had not superseded the CI22 completely. The new speech processor was designed to work at both frequencies and with both data protocols. The new implant would also work with the old communication protocol, although not at the lower frequency. Cochlear's design also allowed its existing speech processor, the Spectra, to be built in a 5 MHz version. As a final back-up, the new monopolar implant could also be used in the previous intracochlear modes. Systematically, eliminating each new aspect at a time, Cochlear could identify the sources of the difficulties although not always their specific details. It was a very traumatic time for the company. Engineers and managers were frustrated but those outside the company would not have known, except for two trial clinics and a few adventurous and courageous patients.

Just as implant development progressed, the external part of the system, the speech processor, developed in parallel. The initial 1982 clinical offering was the WSP – the wearable speech processor. A prototype run of 10 units was produced for a clinical trial. The units had a housing made from a section of plastic drainpipe which was flattened by heating then stretched between two wooden dowels. For the production version, the processor was re-engineered by Peter Crosby into a more clinically usable system, where the processor memory could be rewritten without removing it from the unit and connection could be made without opening the box. These were essential changes if the device was to be a more user-friendly, professional piece of equipment rather than a research device.

In service, the WSP was unreliable. Some of the parts put strain on the solder joints. Solder does not stand up kindly to movement and these joints quickly fractured.

Moisture from the patient's body got into the imperfectly sealed hybrid circuits, since the WSP was usually worn under clothing, and caused early failures. Every WSP sounded different and patients were unhappy when their unit was replaced by a loan unit that sounded different. Then, when their own unit was returned, they were unhappy again.

The researchers at the UOM and CRC continually investigate better ways to code speech. After speech-coding strategy had returned to a minimalist approach when simultaneous stimulation of a whole speech signal using a bank of tuned filters failed, only the voice pitch and the second peak of the speech signal, the formant F2, were coded. Although it made sense, it gave speech a very high-pitched and unnatural sound. It also prevented speech being understood in the absence of lip-reading. The first formant or peak, F1, could be seen on the lips but since it was not present in the stimulation it could not be heard. Telephone conversations would be impossible. The research into introducing F1 progressed methodically, involving tests to ensure that F1 did not compete with or mask F2. From Sydney, it appeared that nothing was happening. Seligman, closer to the trials in Melbourne, could see that progress would take a long time. Why not build a processor which could code F1 anyway? Was there any reason why providing more speech information to patients was not going to work? He started on development of a new hybrid circuit, with support from Jim Patrick in Sydney. The idea had not been part of the original project plan. When the new project was under way, Peter Blamey said to Seligman, 'You're leaving us behind. Peter. We haven't done this work yet.' Seligman replied, 'We'll find out soon if it works and you can prove *why* it works later.'

The introduction of F1 improved patient speech performance, although some patients took a while to adapt to it. This provided a new insight into speech-coding development. Laboratory tests do not always prove that something is working. Patients often need time to adapt, and the only way to provide it is to give them a working device. The new processor was called the WSP3 (the prototype was WSP1 and the first commercial version was WSP2, although it was unnumbered on release).

Providing more speech information was a success but it addressed only some of the deficiencies of the WSP. Seligman, now working for Cochlear in Melbourne, bore the brunt of patient dissatisfaction. 'I was the one who faced the patients when their processor stopped working, soldered up fractured joints, replaced the failed hybrid circuits and listened to their complaints when the processor sounded different to before.' Service staff in other regions were also under pressure. It was time for a different approach to processor design.

At this time Cochlear became interested in Austek Microsystems, a new Australian company. Craig Mudge, originally with the CSIRO, was involved in starting the company. The idea was that Australia should have its own semiconductor design industry which could develop customised chips for Australian products. Silicon Valley companies preferred clients who wanted huge quantities of chips and they were reluctant to do custom designs. Austek had developed a frequency analysis chip for radioastronomy, which was also a good fit for the Cochlear design.

Seligman believed that a smaller, more reliable and more consistent processor should be built on a silicon chip rather than involve the connection of a larger number of small chips and other components together in a hybrid circuit. He put the idea to David Money and Jim Patrick in Sydney. Initially, it was not well received. The chip would require both analog and digital technology. Money, who could speak with authority, with his background at Amalgamated Wireless Australia Micro-electronics (AWM), said that mixed analog and digital chips were a recipe for disaster. Patrick was more optimistic and agreed to get a proposal and quote from Austek in Adelaide. Thus began a very fruitful collaboration with an exciting new and very professional Australian company. Peter Single, who later joined Cochlear, was the engineer and leader in Adelaide and dealt directly with Seligman in Melbourne. The project was managed by Rob Clarke. The chip was designed and built in time and within budget. It worked like a dream and the days of hand-crafted hybrid circuits were over.

Although the electrical side of the replacement of the WSP was going well, the casing for the new processor was not. An in-house design was started but Ron West, CEO of the US office, insisted that the new processor should be designed by industrial designers, not by engineers. But the contractors developed a case design that was overly fragile for something that would be used all day, every day and there were innumerable iterations and hiccups. Even simple things such as the battery contacts became major obstacles. There was intense frustration about having developed a working chip in record time but having no case to put it in. The stress was even greater for the marketing staff who were worried about recent product releases by the competition.

While the speech processor box difficulties were being resolved, Richard Dowell at the implant clinic and Seligman in Melbourne were contemplating the next step in speech coding. Providing the F1 and F2 formants and voice pitch was fine for voiced sounds, but Dowell pointed out that F3 was missing and that the lack of high-frequency information was limiting consonant performance. The competitive Symbion (Inneraid) filterbank device was achieving quite good performance by stimulating on four fixed electrodes. Dowell and Seligman thought that they could improve on that. Why not stimulate on two roving electrodes to present the lower formants and use fixed electrodes for high-frequency information? Thus the Multipeak strategy evolved. It was initially implemented by placing a piggyback box on the back of the case of the production samples of the new speech processor. The box contained four filters to extract the high-frequency sound components.

By this time, the US office was getting extremely worried about the lack of a new offering from Cochlear. After the long wait, the idea that Cochlear would introduce a new processor that used the existing speech-coding strategy seemed like poor company tactics. West appealed to the Sydney head office, which asked Seligman whether the Multipeak strategy, known as MPEAK, could be implemented in the new processor. 'Yes, of course,' was the reply.

As the inclusion of MPEAK was an afterthought, the extra filters required to implement it had not been implemented on the Austek chip. Instead, they were implemented in switched capacitor technology by a company in San Jose called KMOS, formerly Kashtronics. The company was run by Rich Kash, a lively and talented engineer who did most of his work using pencil and paper. He had large templates printed with the parts available on the semicustom analog/digital chips which he had designed, and worked out how to connect them by marking up the paper copies. Seligman made trips to San Jose to work with the competent and pleasant staff. The company premises were basic – staff worked in a shed and there was a minimal front office. The chip was quickly ready and Cochlear released its new processor, the MSP (miniature speech processor), with a new speech-coding strategy. MPEAK was on its way.

Cochlear's first attempt at a behind-the-ear (BTE) sound processor was in 1988 at the time when it was using the Multipeak strategy. A group including Tony Nygard put together a proposal for a BTE processor which could implement MPEAK. However, the processor would be larger than the biggest BTE hearing aid so the group showed the design to the clinicians at the Melbourne Cochlear Implant Clinic. Their advice was that the size was a serious concern.

The project team regrouped and decided that instead of building a smaller sound processor the company should build a better sound processor. This was to be Cochlear's first foray into digital signal processing (DSP). The engineers responsible for it were Tony Nygard, Rob Jensen and Nevil Inglis. The idea was to build a processor that could implement any strategy, not just one particular strategy. This turned out to be a good idea – the company had tried three strategies by the time the speech processor was finished.

The SP5 development was very protracted because Cochlear developed both the front-end and DSP chips. A prototype version was built from off-the-shelf parts, including a sizeable box for the processor and another for the batteries. The software development and patient testing was done with these prototypes.

The SP5 processor, later known as the SPrint, became the workhorse of the company, with a product life of about 10 years. About 30 000–40 000 were sold. The SPrint was the first processor that could use the Micro (CI24) implant's telemetry capabilities. Brett Swanson became the SPrint guru and supported the product throughout its working life.

Around the time of the development of the MSP, Seligman and others at the UOM renewed interest in the use of filterbanks for speech-processing. Filterbank-style speech-processing was being successfully used by Claude-Henri Chouard, the founder of MXM and Neurolec, in Paris. Seligman remembers that, at a 1983 Paris conference, Chouard showed a movie in which a female implant recipient was facing away from a person who sat behind her and read aloud from a newspaper. The recipient repeated verbatim anything that had been read to her. Seligman was sitting next to Adrian Fourcin, the voice pitch guru from University College London, who whispered, 'She's probably lip-reading in a reflection.' He flatly refused to believe that she could do the task without lip-reading. Seligman was less sceptical. It is highly likely that the woman could do the task, as the strategy she was using hardly differs from the strategies in use today.

After the launch of the MSP, Hugh McDermott, an electrical engineer who had recently completed his PhD in the Department of Otolaryngology at the UOM, approached Cochlear in Sydney with some interesting patient results that he had achieved with a bank of 16 filters integrated onto a single chip by Japanese company NEC. The processor was built by Andrew Vandali at the UOM.

McDermott's strategy was similar to Chouard's straight filterbank approach but included a significant improvement. Instead of having the processor scan all filter channels in a round-robin fashion, he arranged it to pick only the six largest peaks. Thus, stimulation that was likely to be masked and not heard, was not presented. McDermott's strategy stimulated at a constant channel rate of 250 Hz, requiring a total stimulation rate of 1500 stimulation pulses per second. He did not retain the voice pitch stimulation rate used by the existing strategy, because he thought that the very low rate was affecting speech performance and that the voice pitch presentation was providing little benefit to recipients. Some could not even do a simple question/statement test (which tests the ability to perceive intonation) or tell the difference between male and female speakers.

McDermott called his strategy the spectral maxima sound processor (SMSP). Seligman liked the scheme and thought about how to implement it in the commercial device. He made two changes to the SMSP. He increased the number of channels to 20, since that was the number usually available using bipolar stimulation in the default mode. Then he changed the order of stimulation from basal to apical part of the cochlea rather than from largest to smallest amplitude channel. McDermott agreed that it would not make much difference to results, and it was very much simpler to implement. The modified strategy was called SPEAK.

Seligman built a big breadboard of the proposed system. The circuit board was about 30 cm square and linked into a tiny piggyback, or daughterboard of an MSP. With this breadboard, the success of the new speech-processing strategy was immediately apparent – subjects started to get better speech performance scores even without any take-home experience. Lesley Whitford, an audiologist working for Cochlear in Melbourne, and Seligman remember this as one of the highlights in Cochlear's speech-coding journey.

Around this time, Seligman visited colleagues working on the SP5 in Silicon Valley. At a dinner, he met George Hansell whom he had known earlier when Hansell worked for Reticon, during Seligman's first attempt at integrating speech processing on a chip. Hansell put Seligman in touch with Douglas Cox, a consultant and mixed digital/analog chip designer. They worked out that a 20-channel switched capacitor filterbank would be possible and could be done with reasonable power consumption. Seligman returned to Australia very excited, and told Patrick that he thought he could replace the piggyback board of an MSP with another board fitted with a filterbank. The rest of the processor, which included the case, the Austek chip, the power supply, the coil drivers and the computer interface would remain the same. It was a quick path to a filterbank speech processor and involved changing only one part, not everything in the system. Meanwhile the official project, consisting of the Micro (CI24) implant and SP5, was still grinding on.

The biggest problem in Sydney with Seligman's new project was that nobody except Patrick liked it. Cochlear had 20 people struggling with a much bigger mainstream project that involved implementing the existing Multipeak strategy on a new implant, processor, interface, new software etc. It was becoming clear that development was getting bogged down, and Seligman's approach offered a very good back-up. However, it was impossible to have another mainstream development with all the necessary documentation. It was obvious to Money that the only way to achieve the objective was to call it a 'research project' which operated very much like the original tiger team. He and Patrick allowed Seligman to develop his design as 'just a research project', totally independent of the company's main activities. The research project had no timeline, project management plan, tollgates or business plan. It had a staff of four, namely McDermott (who didn't even work for Cochlear), Lesley Whitford in Melbourne, a technical officer in Sydney and Seligman. With such a small team the project ran like the wind. In the final stages it needed more varied resources and a lot of the work was done at the SPEAK workshop organised by Judy Brimacombe in Vail, a ski resort in Colorado. This was a brilliant idea. Everyone worked exceptionally efficiently in the morning and went skiing in the afternoon. The eventual processor was called the Spectra and used the SPEAK strategy.

The BTE sound processor has its own story. The company had successfully launched the Spectra and implemented the SPEAK strategy. The SPrint would eventually be delivered, but what did it offer to patients? It provided telemetry, but that was more for the benefit of clinicians. It was larger and used more batteries. It seemed unlikely that another new speech-coding strategy would be developed soon. They thought that the next logical step was to build a Spectra on a chip allowing the possibility of a BTE implementing SPEAK.

The chip that formed the basis of the BTE processor was called Babel, a name used in the *Hitchhiker's Guide to the Galaxy* by Douglas Adams, in reference to the biblical Tower of Babel. In the *Hitchhiker's Guide* a Babel fish can be inserted in the ear and it translates sound directly into brainwaves, enabling its host to understand any language. The connotation of 'fish and chips' was irresistible. Nygard and Daly were major contributors to this project. Seligman and Nygard agonised over every millimetre of the processor's size, remembering the difficulties with the 1988 BTE attempt. The ESPrit, as the new processor was called, was the smallest processor Cochlear had ever made. As late as 2011 it was still the smallest.

The project's single aim was to build an entire speech processor on a chip with power consumption low enough to be supplied by hearing aid batteries. Minimal additional components were to be used. The specification of the chip was relatively simple – the devil was, as always, in the detail. The design was essentially the same as the Spectra, except that it would work with the CI24 implant, which had much lower power consumption due to its monopolar stimulation and the fact that it was built on a single chip. Although the Babel chip development had delays, on the whole it progressed well.

Seligman and Whitford were a little anxious when the ESPrit was first tested on a recipient. Seligman remembers, 'We switched it on. She (the recipient) didn't react at all so I thought it wasn't working. We had to ask her, but she had just taken it for granted that it would work. We continued a normal conversation.'

Although the ESPrit was a success, it did not replace the SPrint. It did not have the capability of high-rate stimulation, which was the focus in speech coding at the time, and was seen as a processor 'with compromise'. Blake Wilson of the Research Triangle Institute in the USA had announced the success of his approach, CIS, which involved high stimulation rates rather than many electrodes, in a 1991 article 'Better speech recognition with cochlear implants' in the prestigious journal, *Nature*. Cochlear countered with ACE (Advanced Combinational Encoder), which combined the high stimulation rate of Wilson's CIS, which used only six channels, with 22 channels to get the best of both worlds.

Cochlear had pushed everything to the limit to build a BTE for CI24 recipients, who had monopolar stimulators using about a sixth of the charge of a bipolar stimulator. It seemed impossible to build a BTE for the older bipolar CI22. However, there is nothing like the word 'impossible' to fire the imagination. Rather than dismiss the idea, Seligman decided to see what proportion of recipients could be fitted.

Statistics were collected on about 200 recipients, on threshold (T) and comfortable (C) levels of stimulation and the thickness of the skin flap covering the implant. The skin flap thickness was important since it determined the power consumption of the RF link. A special skin flap thickness meter was built for this. The team in Melbourne was helped by John Beesley, founder of BWD, an iconic Australian company which built oscilloscopes and electronic instruments.

The next step was to work out how many CI22 recipients would be suitable for a BTE processor. This involved building a jig which could move the coils to varying separation distances. Computer interface circuitry measured the supply current over the range of distances. Using the statistics on the C levels, a synthetic population of all possible skin flap thicknesses and C levels, in their correct proportions, was created. The result was surprising. There were far more suitable candidates than expected. The team realised it had a tool which could be used to maximise the fittable population.

A further step towards the creation of the ESPrit 22, as it was later called, was to build a set of candidate coils for the proposed processor. Each coil was put through the characterisation process and the one that gave the highest fittable population would be chosen. But it wasn't high enough. An important part of the new product would be a controller that could accurately adjust the power to the implant to exactly the right level.

Another aspect was to lower the power requirements of the recipients who didn't qualify. This could be done with bipolar stimulation by widening the mode (spacing between the stimulating electrodes). Audiologists measured how the C levels dropped as the mode was widened, and included recipients who could use a wider mode in the acceptable group. The lower power requirement created by using a wider mode meant that there were only 18 electrodes in use instead of 22, but an acceptable number for good speech discrimination.

With these innovations the number of suitable recipients was increasing but the engineers were approaching a new hazard. The current drawn by the processor was highly variable but the current output of the zinc–air hearing aid batteries was very limited. If a loud sound increased the current above a critical level, the battery voltage would drop and the processor chip would cut out. This would be extremely annoying and would almost certainly mean the device was not a viable product.

To avoid the hazard, Seligman used an approach that involved circuitry detecting battery voltage that was just above the level at which the processor would cut out, and taking action to avoid a cut-out. The easiest action was to lower the stimulation rate. Lowering the rate has a small impact on performance but is preferable to the processor cutting out. It was thought the loud noise was probably not a sound the recipient wanted to hear, such as a train, loud music or other background noise, not speech. Lowering the rate would be by far the lesser of the two evils. When the noise had passed the rate could gradually increase back to its normal level, thus the processor could operate without cutting out.

Finally, the ESPrit for the CI24 ran straight off the battery, without any regulator. This was done in the interest of efficiency and size since there was no space for a regulator and no spare power either. The disadvantage would have been that as the voltage dropped, the power to the coil would also drop. This was overcome by measuring the supply voltage and using the new coil power controller to adjust its output to maintain a constant level regardless of the battery voltage.

With these changes, approximately 95% of CI22 recipients were suitable for an ESPrit 22. The project went ahead, but not without a lot of pain. ABB Hafo, the chip design company, had changed ownership, the staff had changed and the software was obsolete. It was almost like starting again. The problem was addressed by Single, formerly an employee of Austek but by then working for Cochlear. Single, commanding a group called the 'Red Team', got the project back up to speed but it took six months work by 10 engineers. He told Seligman, 'What you did was just a feasibility study. We had to design it.' At times, management does not recognise the importance of maintaining momentum on a project. The ESPrit with the Babel chip could have rolled straight on to the ESPrit 22 with a Babel 22, but the delay in the decision cost the company dearly.

By the time the company acquired the Philips division, Philips Hearing Implants, in 1999 it was time to build an all-encompassing sound processor which was based on a DSP (Digital Signal Processor) and was also a BTE. Cochlear had a DSP (the SPrint) and a BTE (the ESPrit), but it did not have both in the one processor.

Advertising literature at the time had implied that Philips Hearing Implants was a new company entering the cochlear implant market. Given the commercial resources of the company and its global reach, it could have been a threat to Cochlear but no Philips launch eventuated. Following the purchase of Philips by Cochlear, Cochlear's engineers were astounded at the revelations. Philips Hearing Implants did not have a new product ready for launch; it had one that was years away from commercial release.

The Philips BTE chip (the CHAMP) was a 16 DSP-core, 32-channel device that was developed for CIS-like strategies and that did not support strategies such as SPEAK or ACE. It was a bit like a DSP-version of the switched-cap filterbank in the Babel chip and it was programmed using an Excel spreadsheet. There was a prototype version of the chip, but the plan was to use a body-worn processor as an intermediate step. The electrode was a totally untried structure using a distributed common ground. The implant had many discrete components (parts not integrated onto the main chip), extra integrated circuits and high power consumption. The software was also at prototype stage.

The Philips Hearing Implant technology at first integrated only partially into Cochlear's products. The 16-core DSP was completely redesigned into a four-core DSP and it later became the DSP engine in the Freedom and CP810 sound processors. There was an attempt to redesign the 32-channel implant chip with 32 current sources into CIC5 (the successor to the CIC4 chip used in the Freedom implant), but the project stalled in 2002 due to budget constraints. The Laura 34 body-worn processor was initially considered as a replacement for the SPrint sound processor. It was to be the first Cochlear sound processor with a graphical user interface, a built-in infrared computer interface and a dual microphone input, but halfway through the project the Cochlear product plan changed and the plans to commercialise the Laura 34 sound processor were discarded. Body-worn processors were on the way out. However, as the Laura 34 was the only device that was ready to drive the Freedom implant during its validation trial from August 2002 (until the Freedom sound processor in 2005) it was used as a research sound processor, together with the Nucleus Programming Environment software which was derived from the Laura software. Cochlear later commercialised a variant of the Laura 34 sound processor to fulfil its contractual commitment to support about 100 early Laura users with a new sound processor, true to the company's 'Hear now. And always' motto.

As mentioned earlier, the best asset from the Philips purchase was the staff, a very talented group who form an essential part of Cochlear's personnel. The R&D group of Philips Hearing Implants became the Cochlear Technology Centre in Belgium. Philips continued to be the developer and supplier of DSP chips for Cochlear's products. Today, NXP (formerly Philips Semiconductors) remains a key design partner and supplier for Cochlear.

All Cochlear's processors are now BTE and DSP. The former Philips operation in Belgium is thoroughly integrated with the Sydney and Melbourne teams and sound processing is conducted almost seamlessly between them, along with the research group in Denver.

Throughout the engineering process of bringing the cochlear implant from a home-grown prototype to a fully-fledged, mature product, was Jim Patrick. His role in Research and Applications, although the name has changed, has been constant and enduring.

The story of Cochlear's early years is an inspirational tale of an amazing group of people. Together they are responsible for the improved quality of life of over 160 000 people around the world, people who would have remained in a world of silence had it not been for their implant. The commercial benefits to investors and national growth in the form of exports, highly skilled employment and R&D cannot be overlooked. The UOM and the Commonwealth government have earned over $10 million in royalties from their intellectual property, which is an excellent return on their initial investment. Ex-employees have led other Australian companies to success and provided experienced mentoring for potential global players in the Australian biotechnology industry.

The underpinning factor that was critical to the success of bringing sound to the profoundly deaf was the collaboration between the enormous range of disciplines, industries and governments involved in the development of this very complex and extraordinary device. In the Cochlear story, a small Australian medical devices company achieved the right combination of scientific vision and excellence, entrepreneurial flair, strong government support and a global market perspective. A world-class company is the clear result.

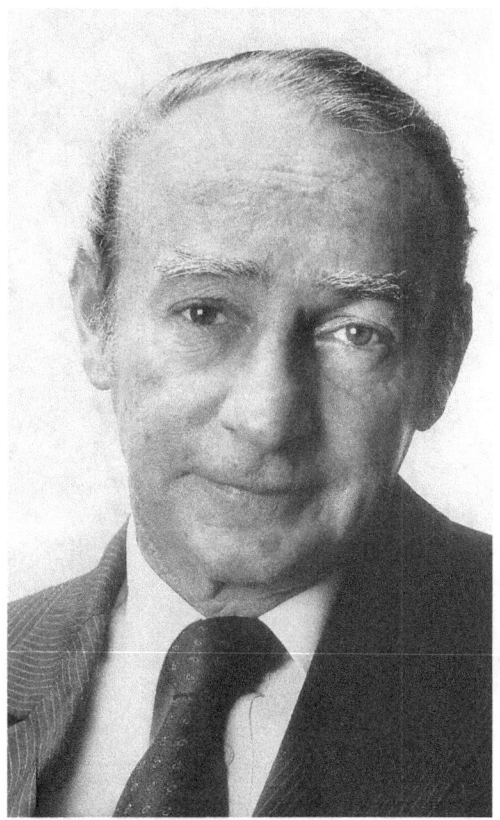

Paul Trainor, founder of Nucleus and father of Australia's medical device industry.

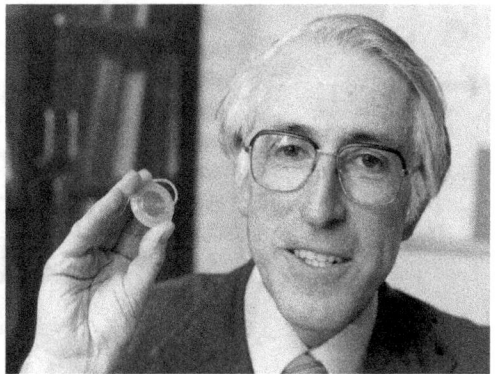

Graeme Clark with the first commercial multi-channel cochlear implant. Source: The Graeme Clark slide and photo collection at the NLA.

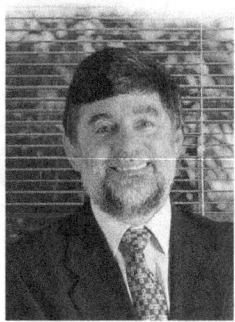

Jim Patrick, a key driver of the Cochlear implant project from 1974 to the present.

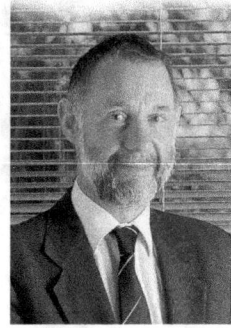

David Money, a brilliant engineer and the first CEO of Cochlear.

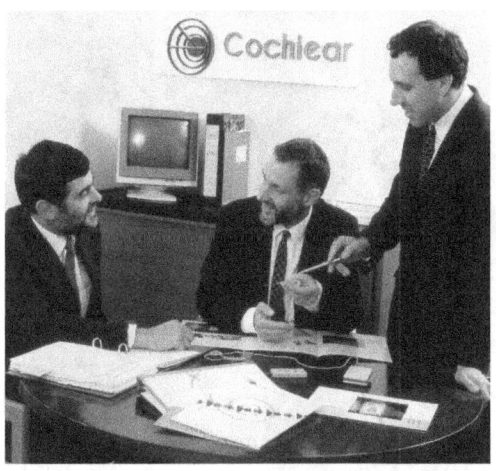

Left to right: Jim Patrick, David Money and Mike Hirshorn.

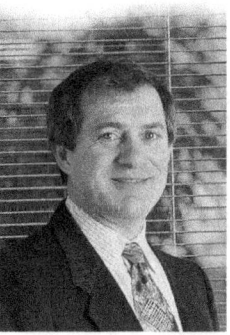

Leo Port, one of Cochlear's first employees, who was responsible for the manufacture of the external components.

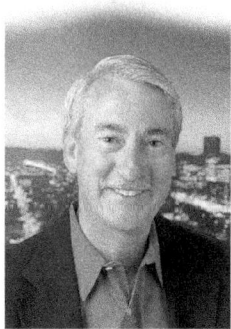

Ron West, first CEO of Cochlear in the USA.

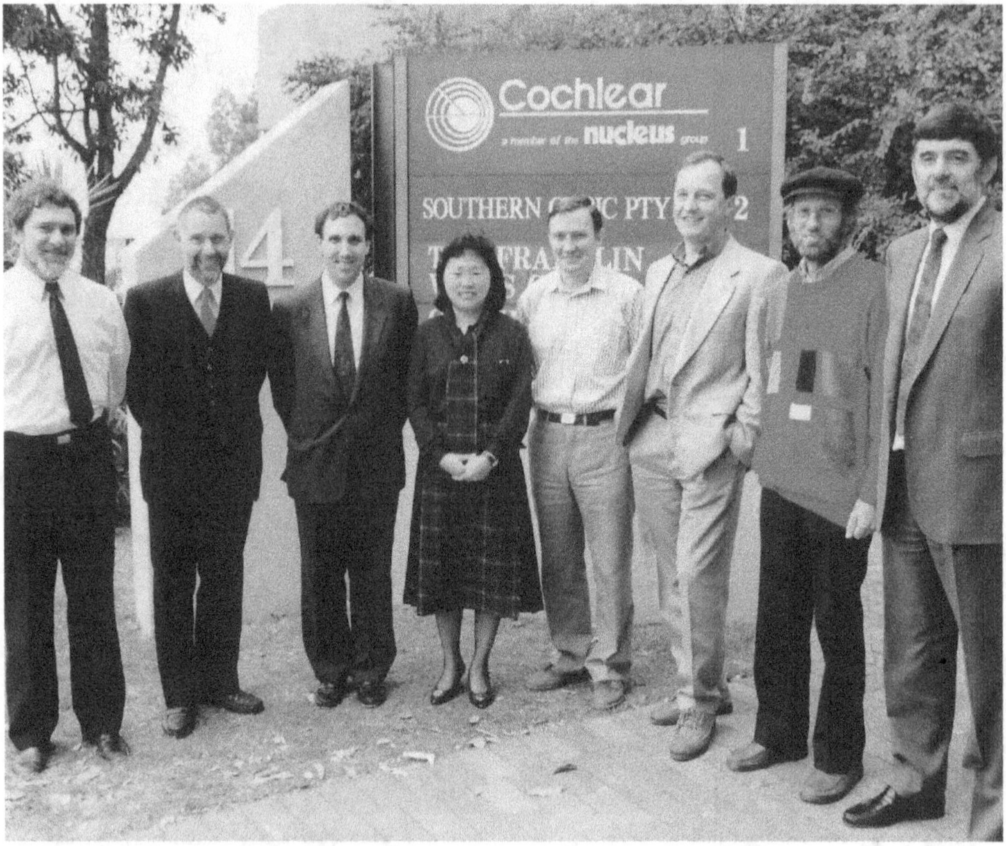

The first 10 years. Left to right: Leo Port, David Money, Mike Hirshorn, Patti Choi, Andy Bursa, Janusz Kuzma, Peter Seligman and Jim Patrick.

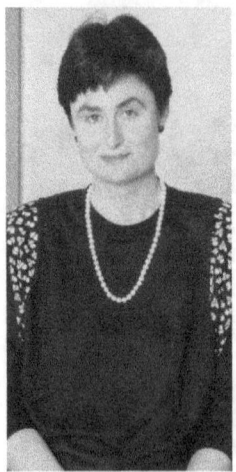

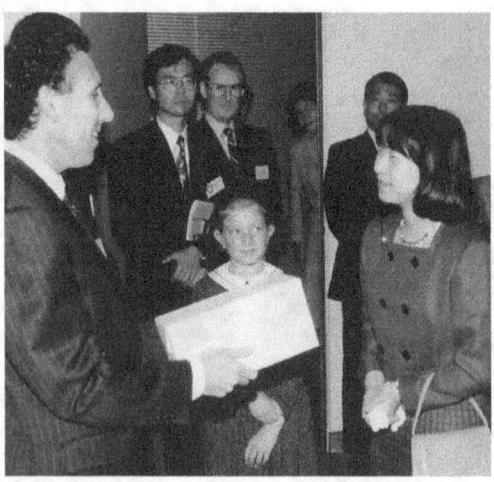

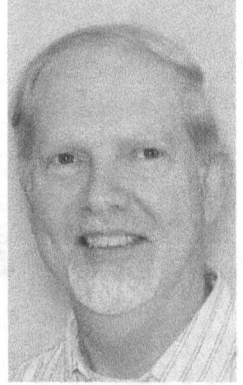

Catherine Livingstone, the CEO who took Cochlear to its float on the share market.

Visit of the Japanese princess Nori-no-miya Sayako (now Sayako Kuroda) to Cochlear. Photographed with Mike Hirshorn and Pia Jeffrey, a cochlear implant recipient.

Hugh McDermott. Although he never worked for Cochlear directly, his numerous innovations contributed substantially to Cochlear's success.

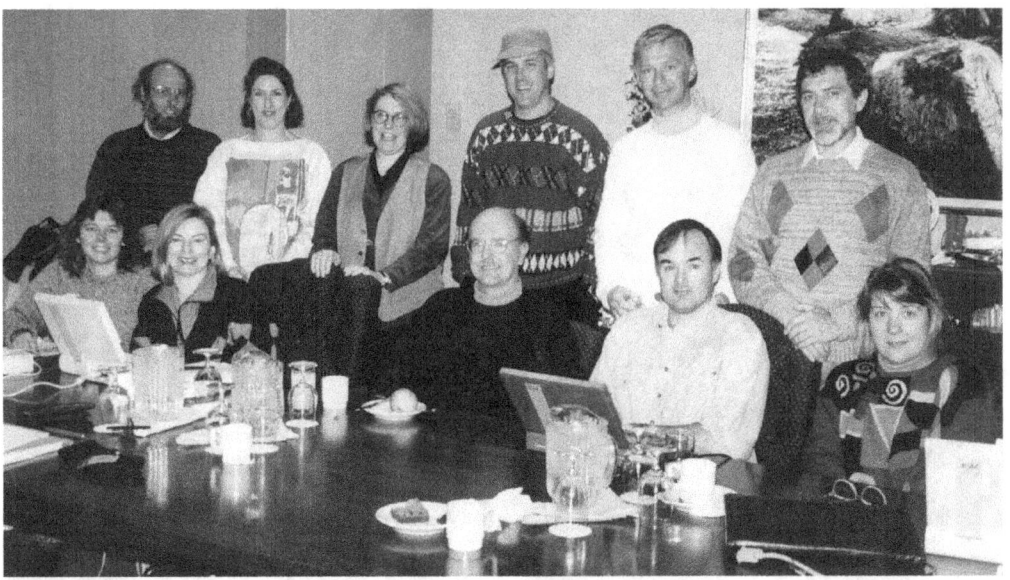

The Speak team. Front row, left to right: Darlene Wolf, Anne Beiter, Steve Staller, Andrew Mortlock and Sue Roberts. Back row, left to right: Peter Seligman, Judy Brimacombe, Lesley Whitford, Mike Wallace, Johan Brinch and Leo Port.

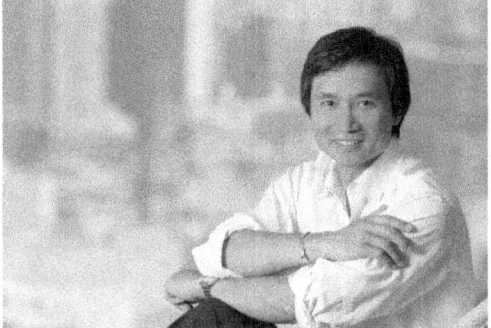

Li Cunxin, author of *Mao's Last Dancer*.

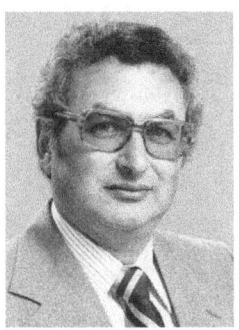

Ralph Tobias, first assistant secretary in the Department of Productivity, Science and Technology.

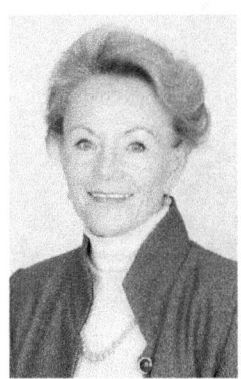

Monika Lehnhardt, the first CEO of Cochlear Europe.

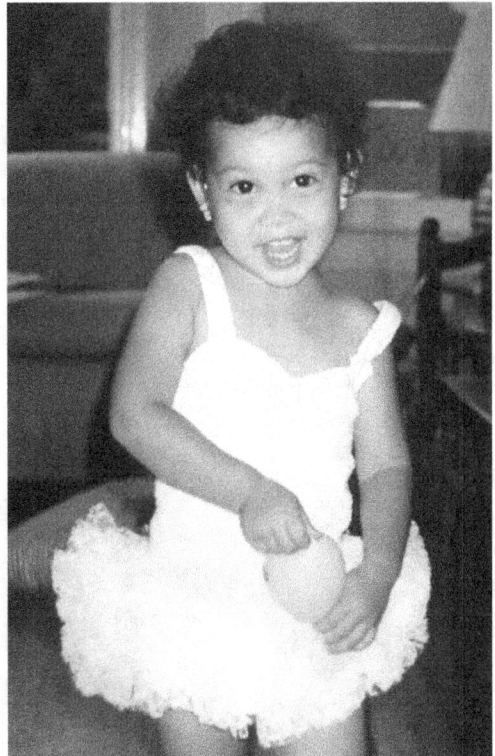

Sophie Li, daughter of Li Cunxin, at age 3. She is a cochlear implant recipient.

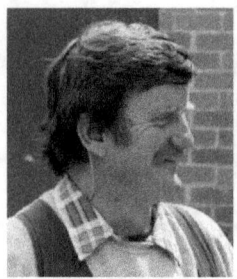

Graham Carrick, the first Nucleus (Cochlear) recipient, implanted on 12 September 1982.

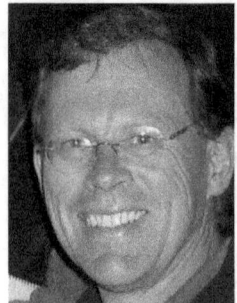

Rob Shepherd, who was vitally important in the safety studies and FDA approvals.

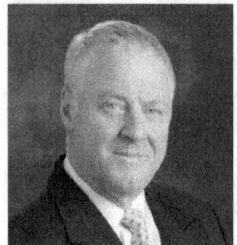

Professor Bill Gibson, surgeon and head of the Sydney Cochlear Implant Clinic.

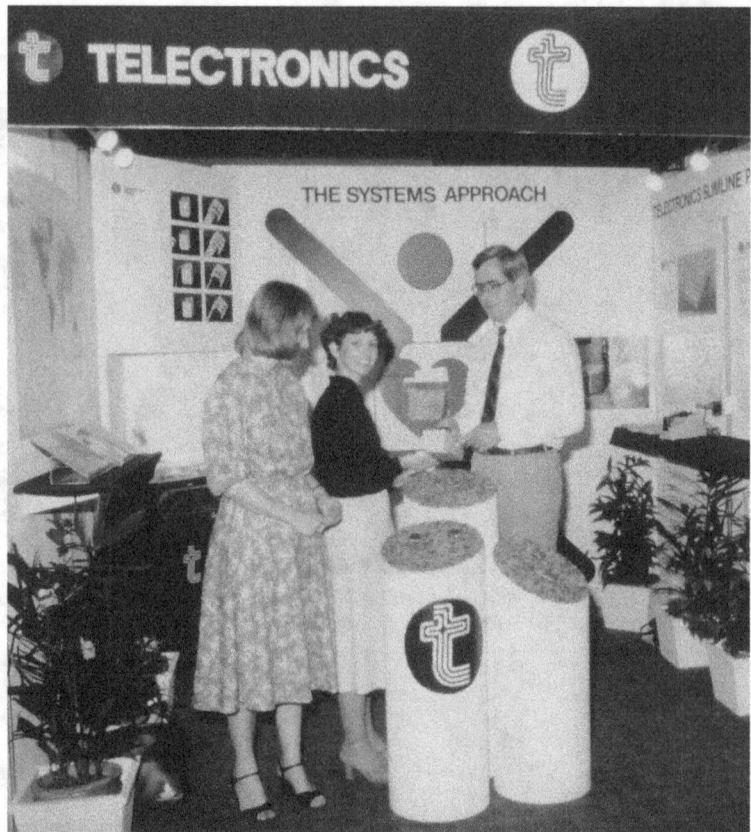

Maria Yetton and colleagues manning a Telectronics Trade Stand.

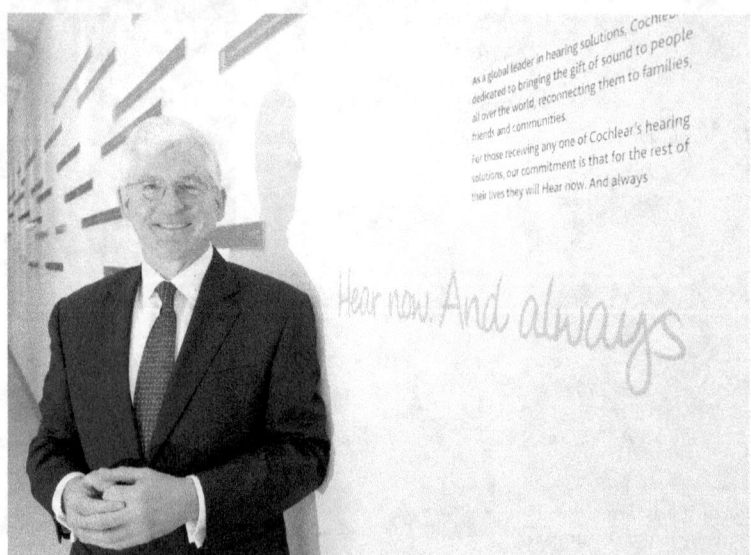

Chris Roberts, the current CEO of Cochlear.

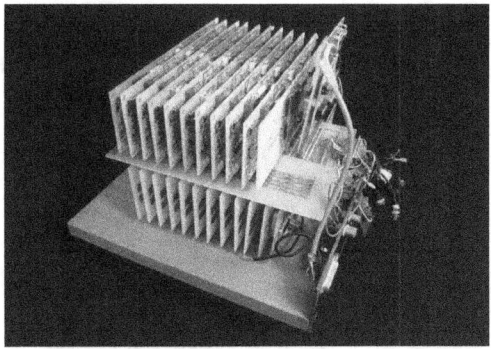

The filterbank of Rod Laird's speech processor which, due to a problem with loudness summation, wasn't part of the first commercial speech processor.

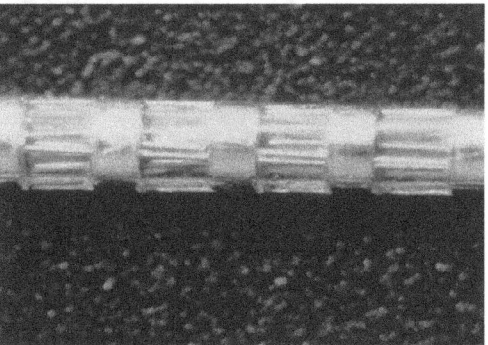

Magnification of the electrode array showing five platinum bands 0.5 mm in diameter and the insulated wires running through the silicone carrier.

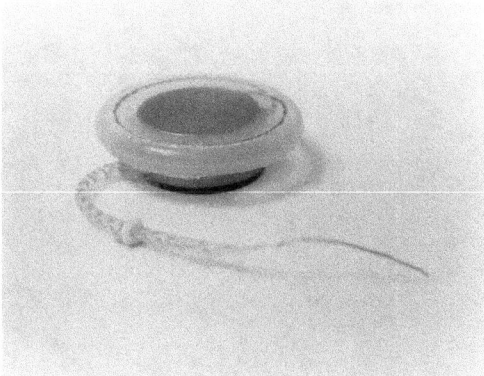

The standard implant, the first commercial release.

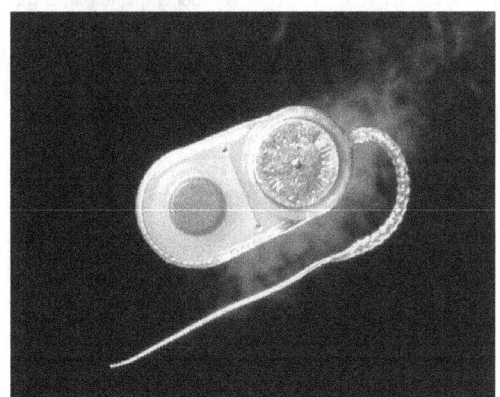

The CI22M, the Mini implant, showing the magnet inside the coil in a titanium capsule.

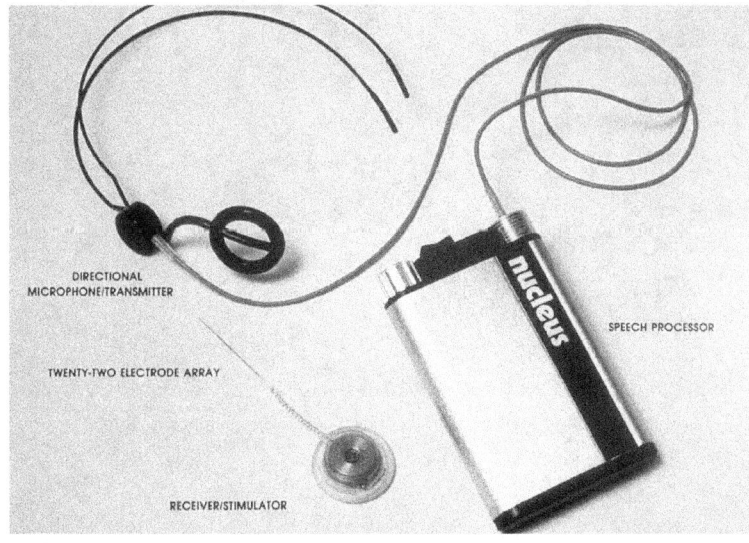

The complete implant system in the early 1980s showing the magnetless headset, speech processor and implant.

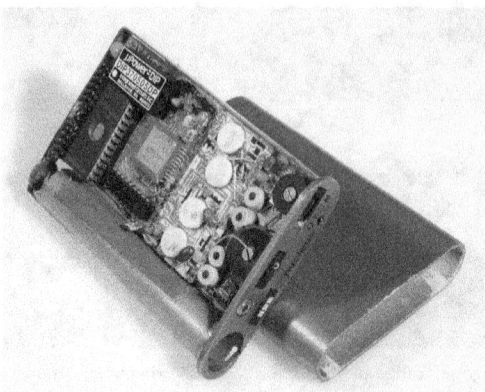

The first wearable speech processor had a case made of plastic drainpipe. The EPROM, encoder chip and one of the hybrid circuits can be seen.

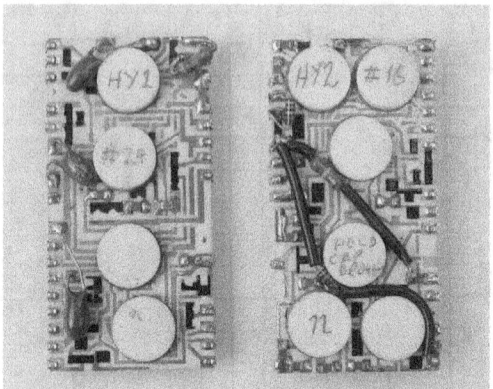

The two speech-processing hybrid circuits showing printed circuitry and the ceramic lids which covered the integrated circuits.

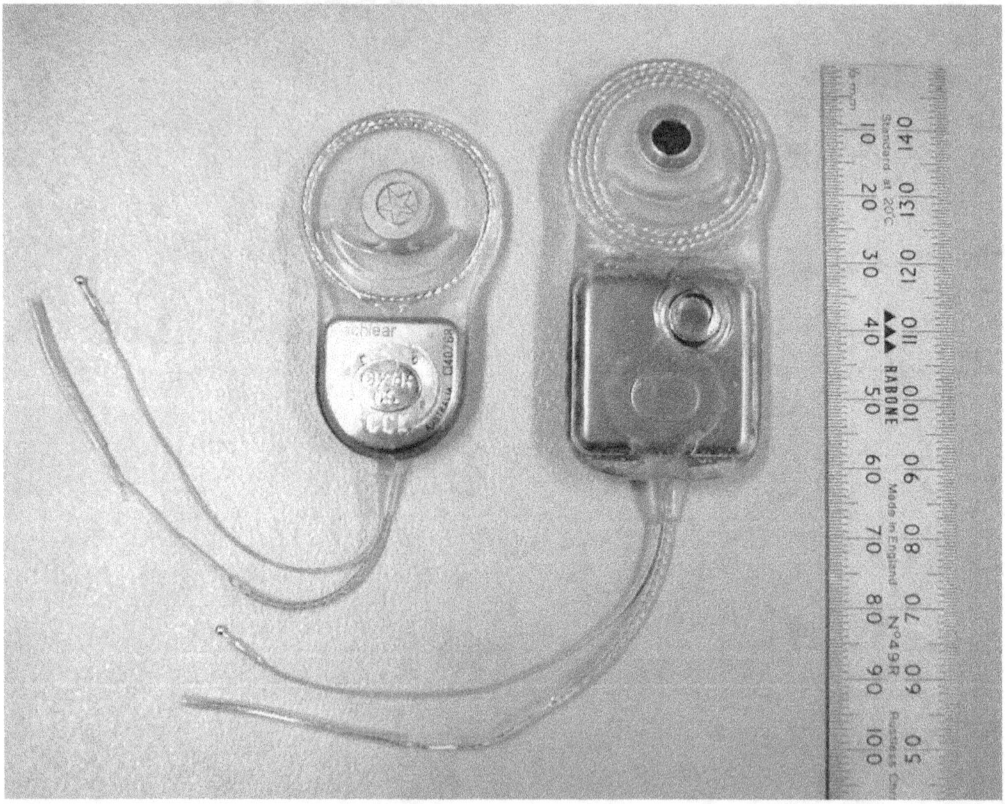

The research prototype for the totally implantable cochlear implant, the Tiki, shown next to a contemporary production implant.

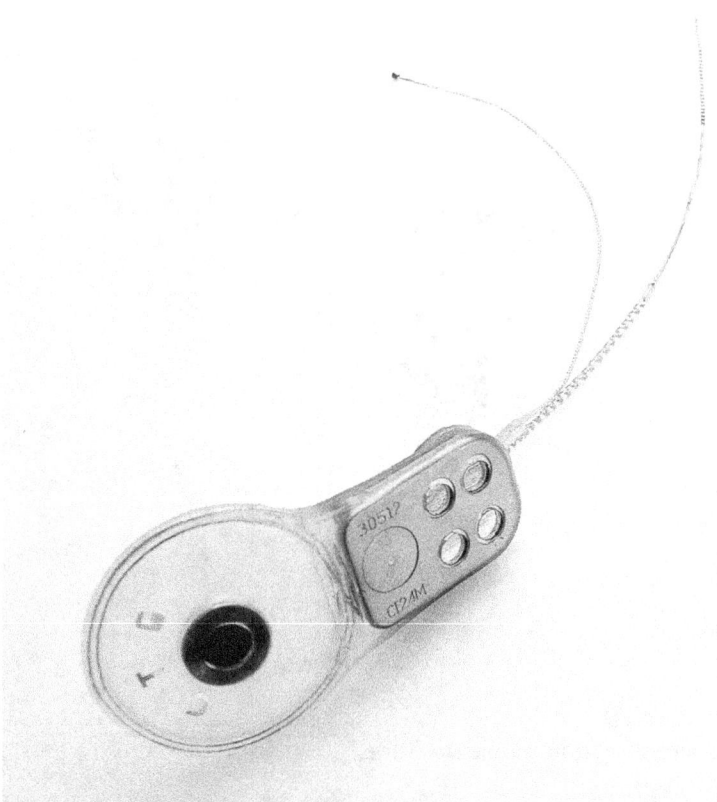

The CI24M, the Micro implant, showing the extra cochlear ball electrode on a lead and plate electrodes on the body.

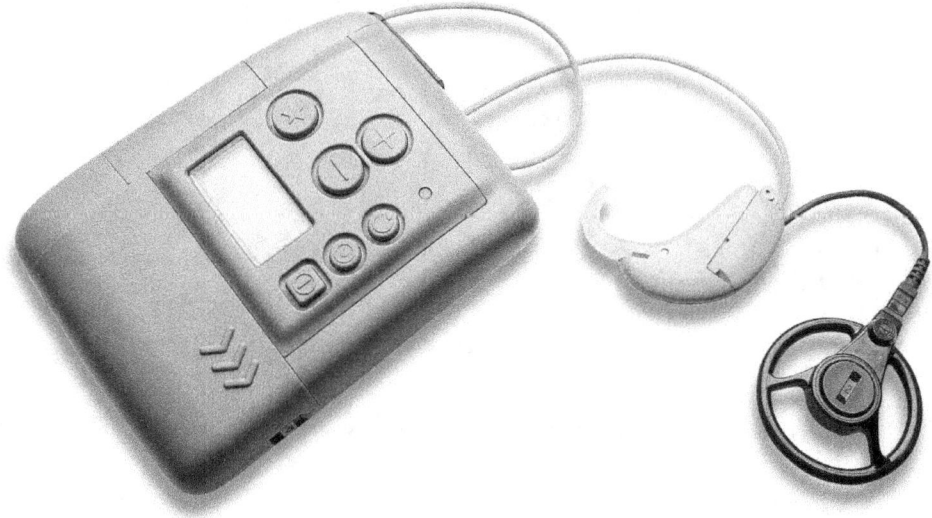

The SPrint. After its long gestation period, it became the workhorse of speech processors for many years.

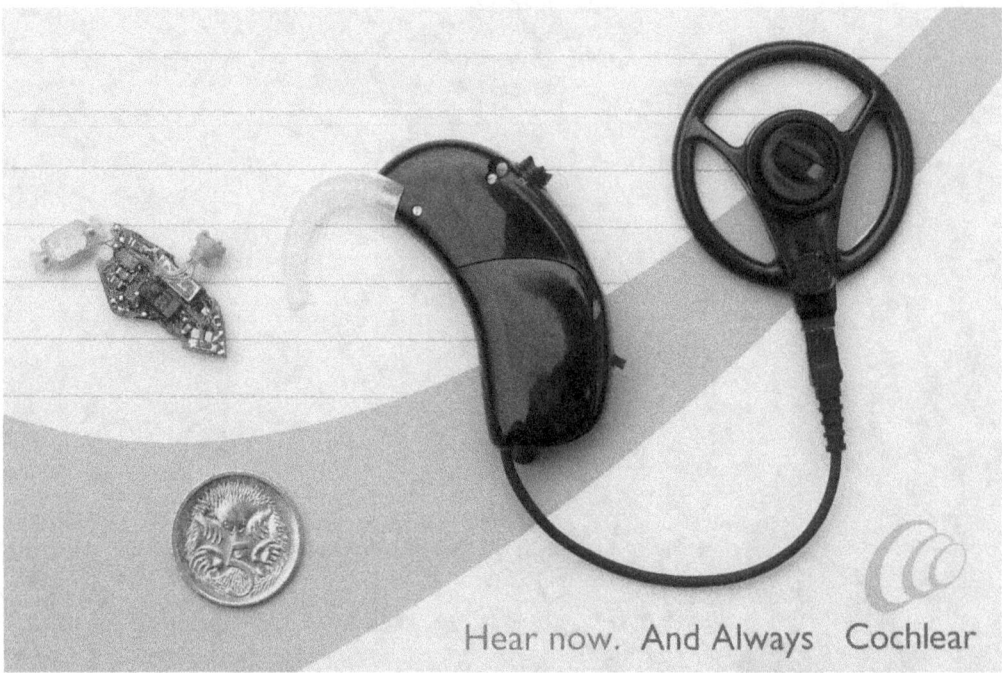

The ESPrit 22, physically the same size as the ESPrit, showing the internal circuit board. Comparison with the 5 c coin shows the size of the device.

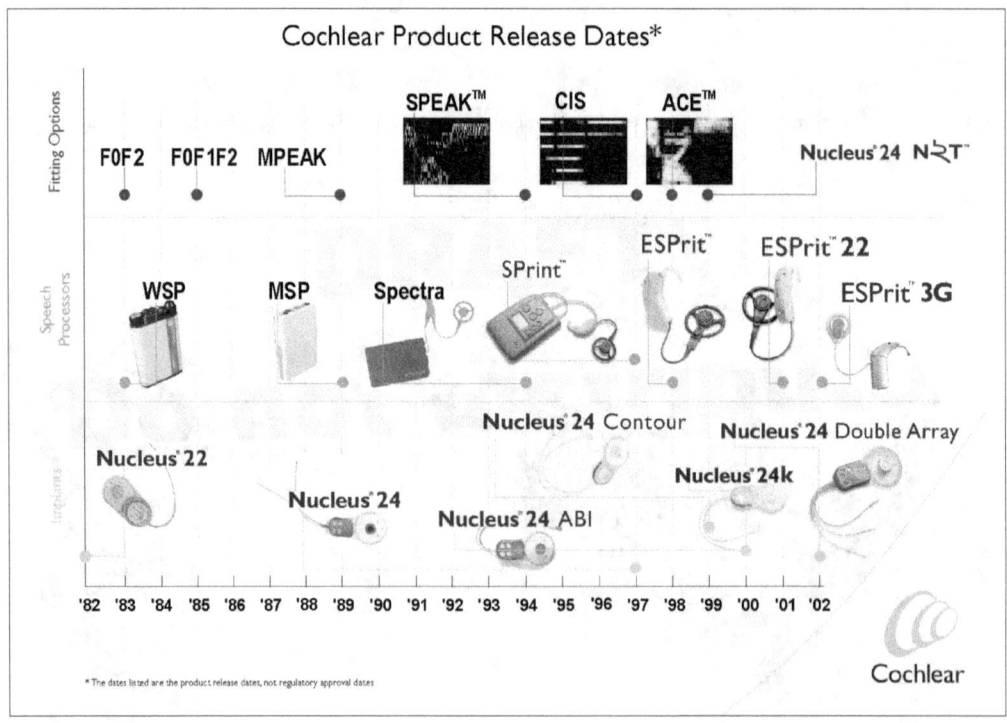

Cochlear products over time. The top line shows the sound coding strategies, the middle line shows the speech processors and the bottom line shows the implants.

United States Patent [19]

Daly et al.

[11] **4,408,608**

[45] **Oct. 11, 1983**

[54] **IMPLANTABLE TISSUE-STIMULATING PROSTHESIS**

[75] Inventors: **Christopher N. Daly**, Bilgola Plateau; **David K. Money**, Pennant Hills, both of Australia

[73] Assignee: **Telectronics Pty. Ltd.**, Lane Cove, Australia

[21] Appl. No.: **252,319**

[22] Filed: **Apr. 9, 1981**

[51] Int. Cl.^{3} A61N 1/30
[52] U.S. Cl. **128/421**
[58] Field of Search .... 128/419 R, 419 F, 421, 128/422, 423

[56] **References Cited**

U.S. PATENT DOCUMENTS

3,662,758	5/1972	Glover	128/419 R
3,667,477	6/1972	Susset et al.	128/419 E
3,727,616	4/1973	Lenzkes	128/422
4,019,518	4/1977	Maurer et al.	128/419 R

Primary Examiner—Wm. E. Kamm
Attorney, Agent, or Firm—Gottlieb, Rackman and Reisman

[57] **ABSTRACT**

There is disclosed an implantable tissue-stimulating prosthesis, such as a cochlear prosthesis, which can not only be implemented in single-chip form, but which also permits great flexibility in stimulation strategy and data transmission format. Only sixteen electrodes are required for stimulating fifteen different sites. Each site is stimulated by a biphasic pulse under control of two adjacent electrodes whose polarities are reversed in the middle of the site stimulation cycle. Although the transmission scheme requires a pulse-width modulation format, the precise form of the format can be varied in order to accommodate widely different stimulation strategies. For example, only a single site may be stimulated during each transmission frame or multiple sites may be stimulated during the same frame. Although only one site can be stimulated at any instant of time, the system cycling is so fast that "simultaneous" site stimulations are perceived. The system is designed for minimum power usage, and its operation is fail-safe in that no site may be stimulated for longer than a pre-set time interval.

145 Claims, 9 Drawing Figures

Front page of the aptly named Daly/Money patent.

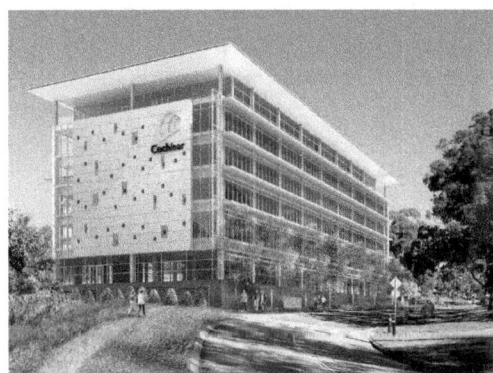

The new Cochlear building, adjacent to Macquarie University in Sydney.

The present invention relates to the design of a package for a cochlear prosthesis as described in my copending patent application entitled "Cochlear Prosthesis Package and Method for Making Same", Ser. No. 402,227, filed on July 27, 1982, which application is hereby incorporated by reference. The connection problem in my earlier design was solved by providing a two-part connector. One part consists of a ceramic plate or sheet containing a number of tubular platinum feedthroughs which form the electrical paths between the internal electronic circuits and the outside. These platinum feedthroughs are inserted into holes made in the ceramic while it is still in the green or unfired state. The platinum and ceramic are fired together and, as the ceramic sinters, it shrinks. The shrinking process exerts a force evenly around and along each platinum tubular feedthrough, with the result that an hermetic, high-strength reaction body is formed between the platinum and the ceramic. After firing, the surface of the ceramic plate is lapped to a mirror finish, and this assembly is then attached to the electronics assembly and a titanium housing using conventional soldering, welding and brazing techniques.

Reference to Janusz Kuzma's platinum feedthrough from his connector, patent US4.516.820.

COCHLEAR PROJECT

We are now underway with this project. We have studied our
aims and goals (see attached) and determined a line of action.

Mr. David Money (who was the first applicant) has been chosen
to lead the project. David's other obligations require that
he allocates one third of his time to the project. The
selection of his lieutenants is vital, particularly for the
early phase of the project. To this end Nucleus has chosen two
competent and complementary people to assist David in leading
this project. They are Mr. Jim Patrick and Mr. Peter Crosby.

Mr. Jim Patrick has joined the group from the University of
Melbourne where he was involved for six years in the Cochlear
Project, being Project Manager for the last three years, while
Mr. Peter Crosby has spent the last three years as Director,
Northern Metropolitan Regional Biomedical Engineering Services.

Other people involved are Graeme Clark, Professor of Otolaryngology
at the University of Melbourne, who has been responsible for the
research leading to the development of the prototype cochlear
device, and his research team, including:

> Dr. Joe Tong, Speech Engineering and Psychophysics
> Dr. Ray Black, Neurophysiology
> Dr. Peter Blamey, Psychophysics

Also in the Melbourne team, working specifically on the Cochlear
Project, are :

Paul Trainor's missive about the cochlear project and the 'aim to achieve the impossible'.

. 2 .

          Dr. Peter Seligman, Signal Processing
          Mr. Grant da Costa, Signal Processing
          Mrs. Lois Martin, Audiology
          Mr. Richard Dowell, Audiology
          Mr. Bob Shepherd, Animal Studies
          Ms. Christine Bunn, Administration

who have the support of four technical staff. The Melbourne
group also has the services of two surgeons, Mr. Brian Syman
and Mr. Robert Webb, working on a sessional basis.

In Sydney the Cochlear team has involved consultants
David Cowdery and Carl Doring in the project, in addition
to recently recruiting the following people :

          Mr. Janusz Kuzma, Mechanical Engineering
          Mr. Trevor Marshall, Electrical Engineering
          Mr. Leo Port, Technical Officer (Electronics)

Via Nucleus we will be coopting Mike Hirshorn on FDA, patents,
and preliminary clinical trials.

The administrative and financial support will come from
Robert Foot/Aileen Wilson/Touchigue Siepa and Liz Noonan.

The plan is to move swiftly to have five implantable prostheses,
together with speech processors, in use with patients by late
1982. Thus we aim to attain the impossible by completing
Phase III in December 1982, that is, to go from the present
experimental prototype to the completion of preliminary
clinical trials.

PAUL M. TRAINOR

28 Oct 81.

Paul Trainor's missive (continued).

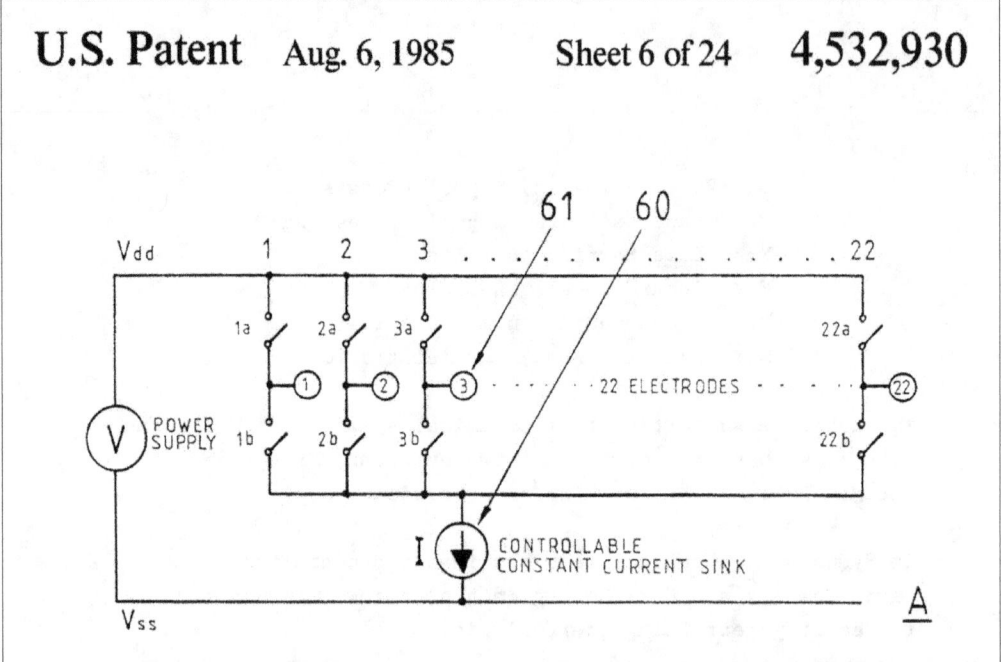

An extract from US patent 4,532,930 including Daly and Money which discloses how a single current source can be used to provide a charge-balanced biphasic pulse.

1985

4.   Research & Development

(A)   Gordon Conference

Jim Patrick and Dr. Field Richards, Senior Lecturer in Audiology at the University of Melbourne, attended the second Gordon Conference on cochear implants. This meeting held over five days in New Hampshire, was attended by some 80 leading research scientists in this and closely related areas. The presentation of our clinical results for 40 patients was very well received, and the preliminary results for our F0/F1/F2 strategy had such impact on one member of the audience that he fell of his chair. In addition to a wealth of technical information, we learned or confirmed at this meeting that:

.   3M has implanted two subjects with 16 channel electrode systems, using percutaneous connectors.

Report of early success at a conference.

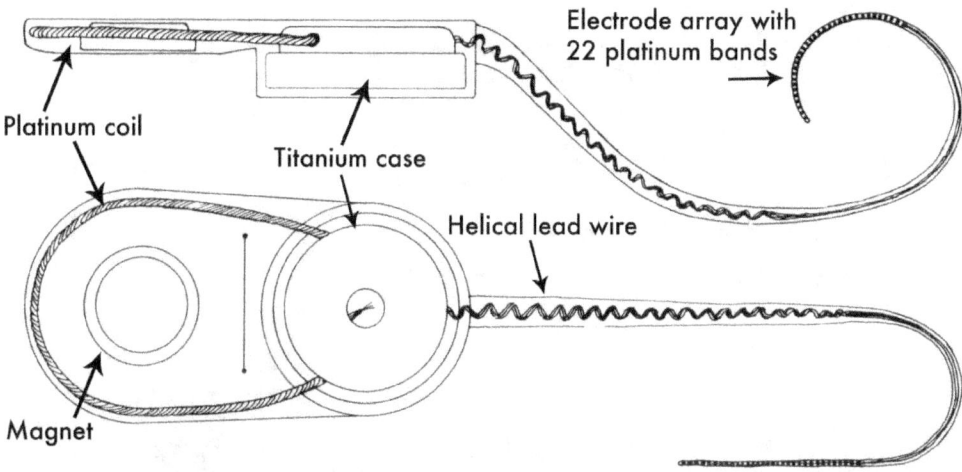

Platinum coil

Titanium case

Electrode array with
22 platinum bands

Helical lead wire

Magnet

The CI22 or Mini implant, showing the major components. The whole device is encapsulated in silicone rubber, which is soft and keeps the parts together.

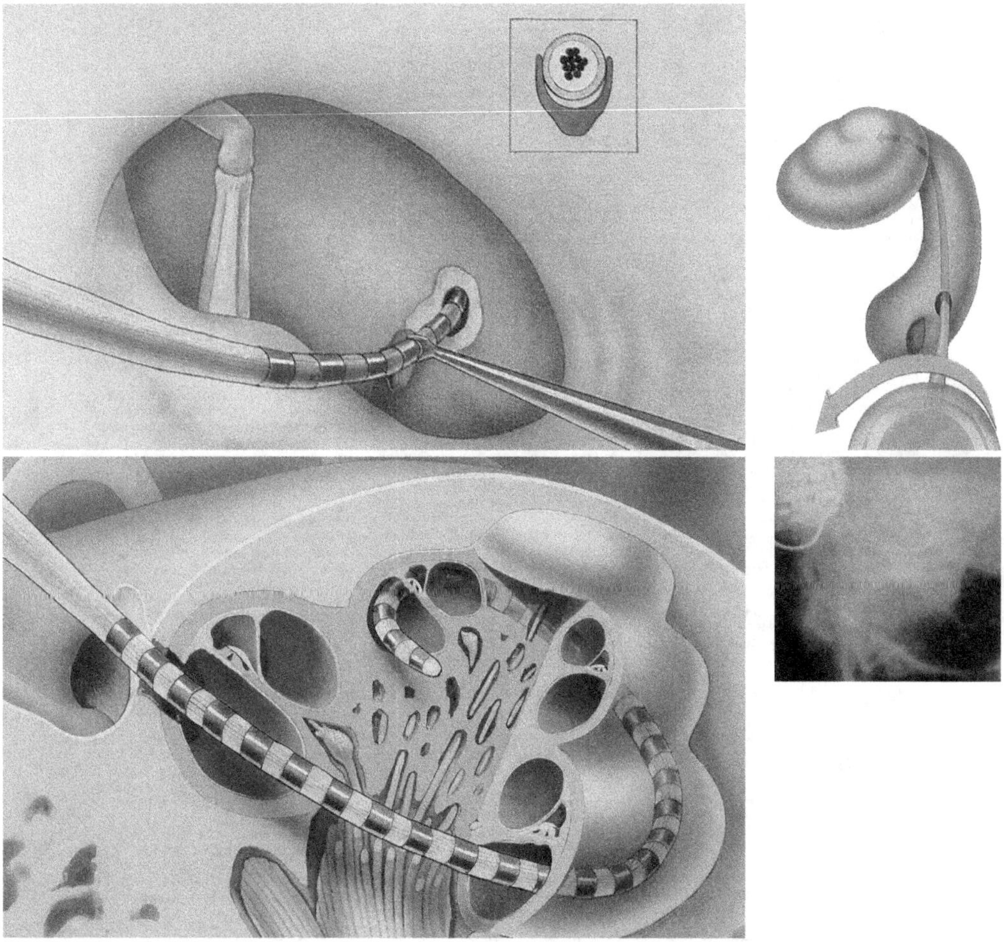

Drawings by Ed Zilberts from the Cochlear surgery manual. Many surgeons from around the world contributed to this manual.

High-tech firm takes on the world

Annual sales of $74m and 800 staff in 42 countries setting the pace

From BRETT WRIGHT
in Sydney

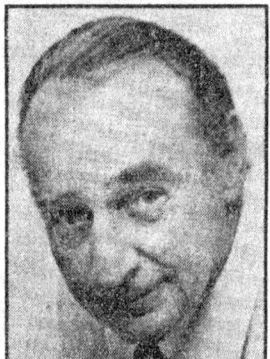

Paul Trainor

THE Australian company, Nucleus Ltd, was a high-technology company long before the term "high-tech" became the vogue. Since 1966 it has been a manufacturer of medical equipment, chiefly cardiac pacemakers, and a leading researcher in electronics.

The Australian Industry Development Corporation, a Government body not known for high adventure and great daring, sees Nucleus as Australia's only established high-technology company, and has recently announced its plan to invest $5 million in the Nucleus group.

According to the corporation's general manager, Mr Don Dyer, Nucleus had impressed the AIDC simply with its ability to survive in a ruthlessly competitive industry and to "overcome some enormous obstacles".

Nucleus was set up in Sydney by Mr Paul Trainor, a former executive of Watson Victor Ltd. It began by making cardiac monitors, X-ray equipment and electronic ignition systems for Jack Brabham. The company quickly expanded into cardiac pacemakers. By 1970, it had begun to export, first to New Zealand and the United Kingdom, and then later to the United States.

The company developed markets in a wide range of medical products, including diagnostic ultra-sound machines and most recently, multi-channel cochlear implants, the nearest science has yet come to reproducing the workings of the human ear.

Today, Nucleus has annual sales of $74 million, mainly in exports, and employs about 800 people in 42 countries.

The company's cardiac division sells about 25,000 pacemakers a year and has captured about 9 per cent of the world market. The entire company has been doubling its sales volume every four years since 1974.

But the Nucleus success story is hardly one to brighten the hopes of Australia's new breed of would-be high-technocrats. In 1981 the company mistimed the launch of one of its ultra-sound machines. It was a mistake that led Nucleus to record a loss of $2.6 million in 1982 and nearly broke the company for good.

A year later, after some hasty management changes, Nucleus made an after-tax profit of $700,000.

Throughout its 18 years, Nucleus has found it tough keeping up with world developments in high-technology — developments which emerge at rates many times that which other Australian manufacturers are equipped to handle.

In 1983 Nucleus spent about $5 million on research and development. The money spent on research by its cochlear division alone totals $6 million since 1979. By comparison, a big Australian building products manufacturer such as Monier, which has a reputation for being research-oriented, spends about $3 million a year on R and D.

Most manufacturers would spend less than 1 per cent of their turnovers on R and D. Nucleus is spending seven times that proportion.

Running a network that sells heavily in 42 countries is costly, too. Last year the company spent $2 million on travel expenses, which is more than most Government departments would spend on travel, while its phone and telex bill is about $800,000 a year, or $1000 for each employee.

Mr Trainor has remained the company's chairman and major shareholder throughout. His warning to any company starting in a high-technology industry is that it is a hard way to make money, especially in Australia where the home market for a high-tech product is not likely to be large enough to justify the industry.

The new cochlear implant is a good example. After 14 years of research and development, Nucleus put the implant on the market this year. Although 150,000 Australians are potential users of the device, Nucleus estimates it will be doing well if it sells 40 implants in Australia over the next 18 months. Hence, exports are an early complication for an Australian high-tech company.

Mr Trainor's other warning is that the marketing strategies behind a high-tech product are at least as important or even more important than the innovation itself.

Nucleus spent $95,000 in 1978 on a survey of the world market potential for the cochlear implant. So, six years before the implant went into production, the

Nucleus Limited.

Offices: Sydney, Milwaukee, Englewood (Colorado), Chatellerault (France), Sao Paulo, London, Cologne, Auckland, Mississauga (Ontario), Birkerod (Denmark).

Subsidiaries: Nucleus Corporation (USA), Telectronics Pty. Ltd., Gel Medical Ltd. (Hong Kong), Ausonics AG (Switzerland), Domedica, Medtel Pty. Ltd.

Workforce: 800.

Turnover: $74.31 million.

Operating profit as percentage of turnover: three.

Ordinary shares: 15 million.

Net tangible asset backing per ordinary share: $1.25.

company knew it could sell about 90 implants in 1984 and about 40,000 in 1990. This sort of market planning, Mr Trainor maintains, is essential in high-tech.

To cope with the special obstacles of high-technology, Nucleus has developed two chief characteristics in its corporate structure: one is a high level of communication between different areas of the company — hence the big phone bill — and the other is a high level of delegated authority. Mr Trainor says the reasons are, in part, geographical.

"It's like an upside-down multi-national," he says. "We are a multi-national but we live in the Southern Hemisphere. Most multi-nationals live in the Northern Hemisphere where they are close to their markets.

"So a multi-national based in the US has all its control factors very close, whereas we're remote."

By Australian standards, Nucleus has a complex and diffuse corporate structure. It's a set-up that easily can lead to serious problems, such as the ultra-sound blunder in 1981.

According to Mr Trainor, that blunder was caused by the heavy promotion of the company's coming generation of ultra-sound machines, while the existing generation went unpromoted and largely unsold. The cash flow dried up and before long the company was in deep trouble.

"Premature ejaculation," Mr Trainor said. "We were getting a backlog of orders of the new one which wasn't going to come out for a year.

"That's the danger of having a market rep in the field too familiar with what you are doing in your research and development."

Mr Trainor rectified the problem by strengthening the company's financial controls, ensuring that a third generation of ultra-sound machines came out on time, and turning Nucleus "into a more market-oriented company".

According to Mr Ross Harricks, the company's marketing executive, the hardest decision to make in a high-tech company is when to stop your research and development work and release the product for sale.

"You get 90 per cent of the way towards the product but so many of these high-tech companies are driven by engineers and scientists who have the ideas, and they want to go that extra 10 per cent to perfect the product," he said.

Cutting from the *Future Age*, 1984.

Appendix:
Interviewees for *The Cochlear Story*

Kiyoshi Arima

Anne Beiter

Graeme Clark

Li Cunxin

Sophie Cunxin

Chris Daly

Leslie Farkash

Robert Foot

Bill Gibson

Ergad Gold

Mike Hirshorn

Shuzo Kimura

Janusz Kuzma

Monika Lehnhardt (Lange)

Catherine Livingstone

Ian Macphee

Hugh McDermott

Mary McKendry

Dianne Mecklenburg

Neville Mitchell

David Money

Hajime Noguchi

Janette Oliver

Jim Patrick

Leo Port

Chris Roberts

Rae Reynolds

Robert Shepherd

Maria Stafford (Yetton)

Sue Stratton (Roberts)

Ralph Tobias

Ernst von Wallenberg

Ron West

References

Ackehurst S (1989) *Broken Silence.* William Collins, Sydney.

Blainey G (1993) *Jumping Over the Wheel.* Allen & Unwin, Sydney.

Briggs RSJ, Eder HC, Seligman PM, Cowan RS, Plant KL, Dalton J, Money DK and Patrick JF (2008) Initial clinical experience with a totally implantable cochlear implant research device. *Otology and Neurology* **29**, 114–119.

Clark GM (2000) *Sounds from Silence.* Allen & Unwin, Sydney.

Epstein J (1989) *The Story of the Bionic Ear.* Hyland House Publishing, Melbourne.

Gibb M (1999) Researcher interview with David Money and Paul Trainor. University of Melbourne, Melbourne.

Haggard M (1991) Introduction: implants in perspective. In *Cochlear Implants: A Practical Guide.* (Ed. H Cooper) pp. 1–8. Whurr Publishers, London.

Hirshorn M (1993) 'Cracking the Asian market, with particular emphasis on Japan'. Corporate presentation, Sydney,12 August 1993, pp.1–7.

Hirshorn M (2002) 'So you want to change your career? Venture capital'. Presentation to MGSM, Sydney, 30 May 2002, pp. 1–4.

Kenney M (1986) *Biotechnology: The University-Industrial Complex.* Yale University Press, New Haven.

Mecklenburg D and Lehnhardt E (1991) 'The development of cochlear implants in Europe, Asia and Australia'. In *Cochlear Implants: A Practical Guide.* (Ed. H Cooper) pp. 33–34. Whurr Publishers, London.

Penington D (2010) *Making Waves.* Miegunyah Press, Melbourne.

Robbins-Roth C (2000) *From Alchemy to IPO.* Perseus Books, Cambridge, Mass.

Seitz P (2002) *French Origins of the Cochlear Implant.* Cochlear Implants, Vol. 3, No. 2. ISSN 1407-0100.

Seligman PM (2009) Prototype to product: developing a commercially viable neural prosthesis. *Journal of Neural Engineering* **6**, 65006.

Smith B (1999) Cochlear Pty Ltd: early stage financing. *Melbourne Case Study Services.* Melbourne Business School, University of Melbourne, Melbourne.

Werth B (1995) *The Billion Dollar Molecule: One Company's Quest for the Perfect Drug.* Simon & Schuster, Sydney.

Index

www.ingramcontent.com/pod-product-compliance
Lightning Source LLC
Chambersburg PA
CBHW080907170526
45158CB00008B/2027